The Practice of Integrative Medicine

A Legal and Operational Guide

Michael H. Cohen, JD, MBA is assistant clinical professor of medicine at Harvard Medical School and assistant professor at Harvard School of Public Health. He is the author of books including *Creative Writing for Lawyers* (1990); *Complementary and Alternative Medicine: Legal Boundaries and Regulatory Perspectives* (1998); *Beyond Complementary Medicine: Legal and Ethical Perspectives on Health Care and Human Evolution* (2000); *Future Medicine: Ethical Dilemmas, Regulatory Challenges, and Therapeutic Pathways to Health and Human Healing in Human Transformation* (2003); and *Healing at the Borderland of Medicine and Religion* (2006). He is also principal in the law offices of Michael H. Cohen, and served as consultant to the Institute of Medicine Committee on Complementary and Alternative Medicine Use by the American Public.

Mary Ruggie, PhD is professor of public policy at the Kennedy School of Government, Harvard University. She is the author of *Marginal to Mainstream: Alternative Medicine in America* (2004). She speaks widely on sociological issues concerning complementary and alternative medicine (CAM) therapies, and has published several scholarly books on comparative social policies and comparative health policy.

Marc S. Micozzi, MD, PhD is a physician-anthropologist who has worked to create science-based tools for the health professions to be better informed and productively participate in the new fields of CAM and integrative medicine. He was the founding editor-in-chief of the first U.S. journal in CAM, *Journal of Complementary and Alternative Medicine: Research on Paradigm, Practice, and Policy* (1994). He organized and edited the first U.S. textbook, *Fundamentals of Complementary & Alternative Medicine* (1996), now in a third edition (2006). He served as series editor for Medical Guides to Complementary and Alternative Medicine with eighteen titles in print on a broad range of therapies and therapeutic systems within the scope of CAM. In 1999, he edited *Current Complementary Therapies*, focusing on contemporary innovations and controversies, and *Physician's Guide to Complementary and Alternative Medicine*.

He has organized and chaired continuing education conferences on the theory, science, and practice of CAM in 1991, 1993, 1995, 1996, 1998, and 2001. He cochaired these conferences with former Surgeon General C. Everett Koop in 1996 and with Dr. Dean Ornish in 1998.

In 2002, he became founding director of the Policy Institute for Integrative Medicine in Washington, DC, working to educate policymakers, the health professions, and the general public about needs and opportunities for integrative medicine to benefit all Americans. From 2003 to 2005, he accepted an interim appointment as executive director of the Center for Integrative Medicine at Thomas Jefferson University in Philadelphia. He is presently a senior fellow of the Health Studies Collegium, and serves as adjunct professor at the University of Pennsylvania in Philadelphia and on the adjunct faculty at Georgetown University School of Medicine in Washington, DC.

The Practice of Integrative Medicine

A Legal and Operational Guide

Michael H. Cohen, JD, MBA,
Mary Ruggie, PhD,
and
Marc S. Micozzi, MD, PhD

SPRINGER PUBLISHING COMPANY

New York

Springer Publishing Company, LLC
11 West 42nd Street
New York, NY 10036

Acquisitions Editor: Sheri W. Sussman
Managing Editor: Mary Ann McLaughlin
Production Editor: Gail F. Farrar
Cover design: Mimi Flow
Composition: Publishers' Design and Production Services, Inc.

07 08 09 10 / 5 4 3 2 1

Library of Congress Cataloging-in-Publication Data

Cohen, Michael H.
   The practice of integrative medicine : a legal and operational guide / by Michael H. Cohen, Mary Ruggie, and Marc Micozzi.
      p. cm.
   Includes bibliographical references (p.   ) and index
   ISBN 0-8261-0307-3
   1. Integrative medicine.   I. Ruggie, Mary, 1945–   II. Micozzi, Marc S., 1953–
III. Title.

   R733.C648   2006
   616—dc22

                                                                    2006049250

Printed in the United States of America by Bang Printing.

Contents

Preface

The landscape of health care and healing in 19th-century American society represented an open marketplace of modalities. Americans could choose from practices ranging from the "heroic" therapies of establishment physicians to centuries-old herbal remedies to a newly emerging form of treatment labeled by its practitioners as *allopathy*. Some therapies, such as homeopathy, were imported; also, let us not forget that many early 19th century physicians were trained in Europe. Acupuncture was introduced to Americans in the early 19th century in the form of English translations from French versions of Chinese classic texts undertaken by Franklin Bache, a grandson of Benjamin Franklin. Acupuncture was included as a treatment for lumbago (low back pain) through the first three editions of Osler's *Textbook of Medicine* in the first decade of the 20th century. Other treatments, such as bone setting, arose on the American frontier where there were no physicians readily available and added to a robustly eclectic practice environment. However, once the nascent American Medical Association (AMA) coined the term *regular* to refer to its members and ridiculed the quackery of all irregulars, a steady decline began in the legitimacy of pluralism. The Flexner Report of 1910 sealed for decades the dominance of biomedicine and the demise of unconventional, nontraditional, unorthodox, heretic, and so on, alternatives.

It is difficult to be precise as to when the use of alternative modalities reemerged. Some modalities, such as chiropractic, continued to expand during the 20th century, despite repeated attempts by the AMA to repress its practice and forbid physicians from associating with its nonscientific practitioners. In contrast, osteopathy gradually entered the mainstream as its practitioners acquired the same educational credentials as physicians. But the reblossoming of most alternative therapies began in the 1960s with the countercultural movement. One term, *holistic*, used at this time to describe what its followers believed was a return to natural methods of healing, seemed to strike a chord that rang through the next few decades of paradigmatic struggle.

As in the 19th century, organized American medicine in the latter half of the 20th century voiced considerable scepticism about the lack of evidence for the efficacy of alternative therapies and about its perception of the potential dangers in using certain of these modalities. At the same time, some followers and practitioners of alternative medicine saw themselves as true alternatives to the mainstream and ratcheted up the rhetoric of disdain. Each side posed the philosophical underpinnings of the other as diametrically opposed to its own. However, sometime in the late 1980s and early 1990s, while some positions on both sides hardened, others began to soften. The softening was swayed, no doubt, by the growing use of alternative medicine by people seeking both wellness and relief, people who were not rejecting the conventional as they sought therapies that they considered complementary, not dissonant. Patients can be credited with nurturing the practice of integration and influencing those who treated them.

Putting integration into practice, however, required a number of preliminary steps and political developments. In the early 1990s Senator Tom Harkin and Representative Berkeley Bedell, both Democrats from Iowa, led efforts in the U.S. Congress to extend additional funds to the National Institutes of Health for the establishment of an Office of Alternative Medicine (OAM). This office was charged with providing the scientific foundation for the safety and efficacy of alternative medicine, to assuage the concerns of physicians. Among OAM's first tasks were to outline a nomenclature for the fields of practice in alternative medicine and to set out a research agenda consisting of both basic science on the mechanisms of action and clinical research on the safety and effectiveness of selected therapies. This research has constructed an evidence-based bridge that is eroding divisiveness and fostering a strengthening link between bio and alternative medicine. It is explaining how both the theoretical and clinical components of certain therapies can be complementary. In 1997 the OAM was elevated to a center and its name was changed to the National Center for Complementary and Alternative Medicine (NCCAM), a change that symbolized a newfound legitimacy and a growth in scope that was energized by a budgetary increase.

Although the term *alternative* continues to be used alongside the term *complementary*, it no longer connotes an antithetical exclusivity between two approaches to health care. Growing numbers of physicians and CAM practitioners now recognize that the term *complementary* is more accurate in describing the compatibility between utilization and acceptance of various modalities that can be used as adjuncts to, but not replacements for, conventional medicine. With this understanding and the practice it evokes, the term *integrative medicine* has emerged. It connotes an active, conscious effort by the health care professions to seek out and sort out the scientific evidence for and applications of various complementary modalities that can be appropriately incorporated into a continuum of health care. Integrative medicine constitutes a new kind of pluralism, one that enables patients and providers of both CAM and conventional treatments to work together to create individualized menus of healing modalities. It offers an ideal that is still far from being realized, however. Continued progress requires continued research on the safety, effectiveness, quality, and appropriateness of CAM, along with improved standards for delivering care. To make integration viable, we also need greater availability of CAM within the mainstream health care system. These two factors, research and mainstreaming, underpin the legitimacy of integrative medicine. Finally, progress could be advanced by research into what still remains a hypothesis seeking more confirmation—that CAM is cost-effective. What little research there is, appears promising.

Acknowledgments

This book was partially funded by grant IG13LM07475-01, *Legal and Social Barriers to Alternative Therapies,* from the National Library of Medicine at the National Institutes of Health.

We thank our consultants who read the manuscript with care and gave us valuable comments: Karen Adams, MD, Richard Cooper, MD, Dean Hashimoto, MD, JD, and David Studdert, LLB. We are also grateful to the numerous physicians and other clinicians, administrators, attorneys, pharmacists and other personnel in integrative care clinics at medical centers across the country, who generously gave us interviews.

Introduction

REASONS FOR THIS *GUIDE*

In the past decade there has been a remarkable growth in the use of complementary and alternative medical (CAM) therapies, which include acupuncture, chiropractic, massage therapy, and herbal medicine, to name a few. Currently, CAM is being introduced into mainstream medicine in the form of complementary and integrative medicine (CIM) and health care, which refers to the combination of conventional medicine, biomedicine, and CAM. How this combination comes about varies enormously, and it raises a host of issues. This book presents a legal and practical guide for physicians and other health providers, hospital administrators and executives, legal counsel, insurers, scientific researchers and funding agencies, ethicists, policymakers and regulators, and others involved in integrative health care. We present the concrete examples of 25 leading integrative health care centers (IHC), describing how they started and evolved, how they make decisions about which therapies to offer, how they handle institutional hurdles, and much more. This information is based on the first federally funded study of its kind. The results are of increasing importance to the future of health care.

There is growing consumer demand for CAM therapies and CIM health care among patients and corresponding interest among physicians and other health care providers and institutions. Many practitioners and health care administrators in conventional settings require a more comprehensive understanding of the legal and social factors shaping the agenda for, and debate about, integrative health care practices.

Among the issues are the following:

- The medical evidence concerning CAM therapies is rapidly growing and in flux.

- Liability concerns are especially prevalent among practitioners and institutions.
- Regulation is rapidly changing.
- Most practitioners and institutions lack consensus regarding criteria for recommending use or avoidance of dietary supplements and other CAM therapies.
- Most CAM services are not reimbursed by third-party payment, yet are demanded by patients nonetheless.
- Many integrative health care centers appear to be physically and functionally separated from the rest of the academic medical center, with a kind of psychic gulf between their personnel and affiliated practitioners and administrators elsewhere within their hospital and academic medical center settings.

No literature adequately addresses the many obstacles to the task of developing integrative health care centers.

Our audience includes:

- *Physicians.* Doctors increasingly are being asked to recommend CAM therapies or refer patients to CAM practitioners. As medical journals continue to publish survey data, showing that more than two-thirds of the American public uses CAM therapies, physicians have an increasing need to become familiar with legal and practical issues concerning CAM therapies. Thus, the book has information required not only for physicians offering CAM therapies or affiliating with CAM practitioners in integrative care, but also for mainstream physicians who are increasingly asked to advise on use or avoidance of CAM therapies.

- *Health care providers.* Health care providers, nurses, and psychologists, as well as CAM practitioners, chiropractors, acupuncturists, and massage therapists, must know the legal and practical issues that arise when integrating conventional medicine with CAM therapies. Many nurses, for example, practice therapeutic touch or see patients who want to discuss their use of herbs. A number of acupuncturists receive referrals from physicians, who require their input. All groups will find this book indispensable.

- *Hospitals.* Within the hospital, health care executives, hospital administrators, directors of integrative health care centers or departments, human resources professionals, pharmacists, and others need to respond to patient (and physician) interest in providing CAM therapies within the hospital or health care center. In addition, physicians who are involved in committees for privileging and credentialing, medication (and herbal) use, pharmacy, formulary, safety, and otherwise involved in institutional policy design and approval will require this book.

- *Attorneys.* With the burgeoning use of CAM therapies, litigators and trial lawyers involved in medical malpractice, attorneys representing CAM practitioners in administrative, regulatory, and licensure proceedings, and corporate and hospital lawyers advising health care professionals and institutions need to become familiar with legal issues particular to this area.

- *Researchers and funding agencies.* It is incumbent on scientific investigators and funding agencies for CAM research to understand the institutional, political, and legal developments that are emerging as integrative health care unfolds. Such information should assist in setting funding priorities, evaluating proposals, and determining if and how research information becomes translated into integrative health care settings.

- *Professional organizations.* Medical societies and professional organizations in medicine, acupuncture, chiropractic, nursing, and other health professions increasingly must help their membership with cutting-edge clinical, institutional, and legal issues in integrative care.

- *Health care educators and scholars.* While the book is presented as a practical guide, complementing theory with many concrete examples, ample references and readable discussion will be of interest to educators in medicine, public health, health care policy, and ethics, analyzing the appropriate role of these therapies in health care practice.

This text offers analysis of a relatively new field of study, namely, the integration of conventional care with the best, evidence-based approaches to CAM therapies. It presents a critical review of the key issues and problems health care institutions face in creating integrative health care. Novel issues include the role of legal and regulatory mechanisms such as informed consent, credentialing, and malpractice liability; how these affect an institution's view of the viability of integrative strategies for care; and the role of cultural authority and how it influences the ways institutions respond to new approaches to treatment.

PRACTICAL TOOLS INSIDE

This text is a practical guide, not just a policy think-piece. We include narrative case studies because we believe there are teachings in the narratives—how individual stories both coalesce to form common themes, yet expose individual and localized creative efforts. The book also offers, among others, the following practical tools:

- Case studies of how integrative health care centers have developed in representative institutions

- Commentary and analysis
- Model strategies for overcoming legal and institutional obstacles
- Suggested policy guidelines for health care institutions
- Supplementary information that will help institutions and their integrative health care centers develop
  - o Credentialing standards and procedures for CAM practitioners to serve as members of the clinical team within an integrative health care setting
  - o Appropriate policies to minimize malpractice risk exposure in integrative health care practices
  - o Guidelines regarding use of herbal products and other dietary supplements

In summary, this text provides the necessary information to help clinicians, health care institutions, attorneys, insurers, researchers, and funding institutions understand how to navigate and shape the institutional, political, economic, social, and legal infrastructure and to develop integrative health care centers together with the legally defensible delivery of health care within these centers. Integrative medicine is a growing trend in U.S. health care. This book addresses a rapidly expanding segment of the market for legal and practical information among the key players in the business of health care.

THE BOOK'S ORGANIZATION

Chapter 1 ("Issues in Integrative Medicine") and chapter 2 ("A Changing Health Care Market") provide an overview of the ways in which the rapid growth of CAM therapies poses a significant challenge to medicine and the culture of health care in the United States. Chapter 1 introduces the terminology used in the field to describe these therapies and the philosophical backgrounds (paradigms) on which they are based. A discussion follows about how the workforce of various practitioners influences use, availability, and potential for integration into the health care system. Chapter 2 describes how the rule of biomedicine created a split into two camps, conventional and CAM, when the latter reappeared in the fourth quarter of the 20th century. It elaborates the way nomenclature changes, from *alternative* to *complementary* to *integrative*, that have mirrored increasing legal, medical, legislative, and institutional legitimacy accompanying clinical integration of these therapies. The chapter also discusses our research methods and limitations.

Chapter 3 ("Assessing the Landscape") introduces the major legal and institutional barriers to integrative health care. It describes the primary components of the legal and regulatory structure governing the integration

of CAM therapies into conventional clinical care. This chapter also introduces the sociology of organizations, science, and professions, and describes how insights from these fields can enrich our understanding of the process of integration, with application to the key institutional obstacles and internal politics that physicians and leaders of centers have faced.

Chapter 4 ("Starting Up and Growing") describes how the centers in our review began and evolved. Two issues have been critical: financing and nonfinancial support. This chapter guides readers through the various survival strategies the centers adopted (including the role of health insurance and research support in securing viability and legitimacy) and evaluates the extent to which various strategies can be effective. We look at such factors as initial and present funding arrangements, size and scope of clinical practice, methods of delivering care, and working relations within the clinics and with hospital administrators and physicians.

Chapter 5 ("Getting Through the Door") provides information that will help health care institutions develop credentialing standards and procedures for CAM practitioners as members of the integrative team. This chapter includes case studies and our analyses of them. We summarize some of the strategies used by leading institutions to credential such providers as acupuncturists, chiropractors, massage therapists, naturopathic physicians, and various mind–body providers. The chapter also evaluates current controversies and challenges faced by credentialing committees, centers, and executives at institutions pioneering integrative health care.

Chapter 6 ("Staying Afloat") addresses the issue of potential malpractice liability, one of the greatest fears and obstacles to clinical integration of CAM therapies. This chapter provides information to help develop appropriate policies and procedures to minimize malpractice risk in integrative health care practices. The content critically reviews and analyzes the relevant literature, offers narratives from interviews, and summarizes some of the liability management strategies used. The focus is on physician liability, CAM practitioner liability, and institutional liability for either providing integrative health care, advising about CAM therapies, or referring for such therapies.

Chapter 7 ("Empowering Patients") addresses legal rules governing informed consent. There is a trend away from a bureaucratic disclosure process and toward an emphasis on a conversation between provider and patient in which a process of shared decision making occurs concerning selection of therapies (including CAM therapies). Integrative health care also emphasizes patient empowerment through such a process. Yet, lawyers may be viewed as intruders with forms and risk management requirements that are at cross purposes to the therapeutic relationship. This chapter aims to help health care institutions develop a framework for disclosure and discussion of CAM therapies in a way that enhances patient

capacity for decision making and thereby promotes the therapeutic relationship between provider and patient. Through case studies, the chapter offers model strategies.

Chapter 8 ("The Supplements Question") and chapter 9 ("Integrative Medicine for Pharmacy") address the critical issues in developing guidelines on pharmacy and therapeutics committee practices for the use or avoidance of herbal products and other dietary supplements. One of the burning questions in hospital settings, for example, is whether to simply confiscate the patient's supplements on admission to the hospital, restock the supplements (from an institutional herbal formulary), or proscribe any and all use of supplements. Such questions are particularly thorny when inpatients are scheduled for surgery. The chapter critically reviews the regulatory framework for supplements; explores the impact of the current regulatory environment on clinical care; evaluates controversies involving the appropriate role of vitamins, herbs, minerals, and other dietary supplements; discusses the thinking behind emerging policies regarding dietary supplements; and discusses strategies for monitoring quality assurance, adverse events, and selecting appropriate products or brands.

Chapter 10 ("Future Health Care") gathers all our materials to construct models of current centers that will be helpful to those considering the establishment or reshaping of an integrative health care center or practice. We also assess factors behind the success of certain centers, the struggles of others, and offer suggestions for the latter from the experiences of the former.

The "Conclusion" synthesizes our data and themes. The number of integrative health care centers is growing across the country. Despite diversity in their characteristics and contexts, common themes are emerging in their experiences as well as their hopes and plans for the future. As scientific research mounts and correlates safe and effective CAM therapies with specific illnesses and disorders, demand will continue to surge: so will the need for wise approaches when scientific evidence fails to support continued use of therapies that are in high patient demand.

It behooves all physicians, health care professionals, and hospital administrators to prepare now for impending changes in the delivery of health care. This review and state-of-the-art summary of key legal and sociological issues will significantly facilitate nationwide development of model strategies and procedures necessary to responsibly deliver and integrate CAM therapies within U.S. health care institutions. These steps are vital to both research efforts and to the development of models of integrative health care and their clinical applications. Particularly given controversies surrounding research and clinical delivery of CAM therapies, organizations and institutions must learn from each other to achieve effective responsible practices and policies.

CHAPTER 1

Issues in Integrative Medicine

Use and Availability of CAM

INTRODUCTION

One of the major popular health movements of the 21st century is widespread interest in, and utilization of, what has been called complementary and alternative (CAM) and more recently integrative medicine. These therapies are used by a variety of people for a wide variety of complaints in a large number of health care settings.[1-10] Following widespread recognition by the medical and scientific communities of this popular trend, there has been a corresponding movement among medical practitioners, administrators, academicians, and scientists to incorporate these modalities into their existing spheres of research, practice, and teaching. These popular and professional movements are now leading clinics, hospitals, health systems, and insurers to invest more deeply and broadly in integrative medicine from the perspective of clinical practice. Federal and state governments are beginning to address the issues related to CAM and integrative practice from the standpoint of public health and health care regulation.

The dimensions of the phenomenon are impressive. In recent years, it is estimated that there were more visits by the American public to alternative practitioners than to primary care physicians.[1-10] Use of herbal remedies and dietary supplements is now supported by a multifaceted industry in the United States generating tens of billions of dollars in annual revenues. Until recently, American consumers have paid for most of the costs of these products and services out-of-pocket, receiving only limited, if any, insurance or tax benefits, unlike other areas of health care. It is also estimated that the out-of-pocket amount spent by consumers for alternative care exceeds the out-of-pocket co-payments and deductibles consumers make for traditional health care covered by insurance, and this amount has been increasing for over a decade.[1–10] These observations are critical for further studies of health care utilization when considering the roles of third-party payers in the provision of health care. A telling example of change is that one last bastion of traditional fee-for-service medicine resides among alternative practitioners and clients who currently receive no insurance reimbursement or third-party payment. Further, the workforce supplying alternative and complementary care is strikingly small when compared to the current workforce of approximately 600,000 practicing physicians.[11] These circumstances require greater efforts to support further studies on health care utilization and evidence-based medicine to better understand the implications of CAM for health care in the 21st-century United States.

In this chapter, we address the nomenclatures and philosophies that relate to the therapeutic paradigms in practice. We then review the various therapeutic modalities classified under CAM and integrative medicine, their practitioners, and the related issues of therapeutic access and availability, with some models of integration (vs. maintenance of pluralism). Issues related to the need and potential for evaluation of effectiveness and cost-effectiveness follow, along with a review of the special requirements for professional education and public policy efforts in integrative medicine.

THERAPEUTIC PARADIGMS

The rhetorical or poetical question of "What's in a name?" has had profound implications relative to the scientific and cultural acceptance of therapies that are not biomedical. Prior to the 1990s the medical and scientific communities proposed such labels as *nontraditional, unconventional,* and *unorthodox,* reflecting their judgments about the validity and appropriateness of nonbiomedical modalities. However, those who used these therapies chose such words as *holistic, alternative* and, eventually, *complementary,* reflecting their approach to their health care. Alternative came to imply a mutual exclusivity between these modalities and the regular practice of medicine, whereas complementary was more accurate in describing a compatibility between the utilization and acceptance of these modalities as an adjunct to but not a replacement for regular medicine.

In the 1990s a national research program began at the National Institutes of Health (NIH) to investigate and determine the evidence (or lack thereof) supporting use of these modalities.[12] Led by the U.S. Congress, particularly by the efforts of Senator Tom Harkin and Representative Berkeley Bedell, the NIH activity was first established in 1992 as the Office of Unconventional Medical Practices, changing soon thereafter to the Office of Alternative Medicine (OAM). In 1998 it became the National Center for Complementary and Alternative Medicine (NCCAM), symbolizing its growth in budget as well as scope. The research generated not only a growing scientific basis for the safety and efficacy of certain CAM therapies, but it also raised awareness within the medical community about how these therapies could be employed alongside biomedicine. A number of health care professionals undertook an active, conscious effort to seek out and sort out the evidence and applications of various complementary modalities for appropriate incorporation into health care within the parameters of their medical training. As a result of these efforts, the term *integrative medicine* emerged.

Integration has come to mean both the combined use of alternative and biomedical therapies as well as their complementary or interactive use. Sometimes the integration is done by patients, sometimes by health care professionals, sometimes by both. Studies show that many people combine therapies on their own.[5-10] A few of the integrative health care centers (IHCs) in our study simply provide patients with the names of CAM practitioners in the community; some patients prefer to make decisions about their use of CAM on their own.[13] However, many centers, especially those that employ CAM practitioners, attempt to involve physicians, CAM practitioners, and patients in consultations at the least, if not joint decision making about optimal choices of therapies. To the extent possible, these decisions are based on the evidence produced first by the NIH-funded studies on safety and efficacy and, second, by social scientific and health outcomes research. This evidence is being published in peer-reviewed journals. At present, it is limited in both quantity and quality. We need much more research; we also need improved standards for establishing the evidence base for the safety, effectiveness, quality, and appropriateness of CAM. The more integrative health care providers know about CAM and about how CAM complements biomedicine, the more they will be able to enhance consumer choice.

To make integration viable, we also need greater availability of CAM within the mainstream health care system. The present, relatively limited, workforce of complementary/alternative medical practitioners[11] may suggest that more appropriate care will be provided to more people through continued integration into the mainstream health care system. In this view, integration would be an improvement over what has often been the situation for consumers with an uncoordinated landscape of different practices, each vying for primacy within as yet incompletely defined, articulated, and accepted evidence-based scopes of practice.

There is a general value to society for the continued existence of pluralism among healing choices for consumers. A few studies are demonstrating that CAM can be cost-effective.[14,15] Beyond economic considerations is the contribution CAM can make to the healing process. Most important for our purposes are studies demonstrating how CAM complements biomedical treatment, facilitating healing in a more positive manner than when biomedicine alone is used. For instance, mind-body therapies reduce pain and tension during early recovery from open heart surgery.[16] When heart patients are trained in meditation, their stress is reduced, improving their rehabilitation progress.[17] The literature is replete with such examples.

THERAPEUTIC MODALITIES

Many of the modalities used in CAM can be seen as existing along a continuum together with conventional medicine. It is useful and instructive to arrange these techniques from least invasive to most invasive. Consider, for instance, a continuum that ranges from meditation, talk therapies, bioenergetic manipulation, massage, physical manipulation, insertion and ingestion to injection, and minor and major surgery. The beginning of the continuum involves CAM therapies and the end involves biomedicine. However, within the continuum, there is overlap between CAM and biomedicine.

For instance, psychiatry, which uses both talk therapies and ingestion, can be considered as having one foot in CAM, another in biomedicine. Both CAM and biomedicine employ therapies that involve insertion and ingestion. Some CAM therapies, such as traditional Chinese medicine (TCM), involve a variety of treatments, such as bioenergy (qi), manipulation (tui na, Qi Gong), insertion (acupuncture needles), and ingestion (herbs and foods) for medicinal purposes. Ayurvedic medicine and Native American Indian practices, among others, were also classified by the OAM as systems of medical practice because they incorporate various techniques. Naturopathy is interesting in that it was traditionally limited to a so-called nature cure following a Hippocratic emphasis on "airs, waters, and places," foods, and herbs. However, contemporary naturopathic medicine consciously incorporates training in and utilization of a large number of recognized healing techniques, which are consolidated into systems of formalized neoeclectic medicine. Furthermore, individual practitioners within one system of naturopathic care may create their own forms of eclecticism by incorporating the use of other healing modalities from outside that system. Similarly, some physicians or chiropractors have begun to use acupuncture.

Individual techniques practiced in a manner that is removed from the traditional system of care, called *formulary approaches*, are becoming more common. For example, in the traditional practice of Chinese medicine, as may be found in China or in the Chinatowns of the urban United States, the client generally seeks the services of an acupuncturist who uses formulary approaches learned from generations of forefathers. Chinese practitioners may wish to incorporate herbs, manipulation, or other remedies for the treatment of a medical condition. Meanwhile, in the United States, a licensed physician in a number of states may attend a six-week course in acupuncture and become a licensed acupuncturist. Research shows that this kind of acupuncture, provided by the physician on a formulary basis, is effective and may in fact meet cultural expectations better for the average American when delivered by a practitioner in a white coat in an antiseptic clinic than what might be experienced with the delivery of care in Chinatown.[18] Other kinds of formulary approaches practiced in the United States today include manual and manipulative therapists who incorporate for therapeutic purposes herbal and nutritional remedies, classified in the United States today as dietary supplements.

THERAPEUTIC ACCESS AND AVAILABILITY

Use of and access to CAM services varies across the United States in accordance with the existence, numbers, and location of (1) practitioners trained (and licensed, where applicable) to provide these services, and (2) practice settings, such as clinics, hospitals, academic medical centers, and health care systems and networks, as well as individual practices, which have existed and often thrived independent of the mainstream health care system. As a result of this diversity, integration involves a number of issues related to local resources and culture.

Workforce

Given the dimensions of the movement, it is often striking how few so-called alternative providers presently exist relative to the mainstream medical workforce. Manual and manipulative therapies are relatively well represented with approximately 100,000 massage therapists and more than 50,000 licensed chiropractors. There are approximately 25,000 osteopaths, with perhaps fewer than one-quarter of them maintaining a practice in manipulative therapy. Manipulative therapy is also relatively well regulated, with licensure for chiropractic in all 50 states and the District of Columbia (DC) and accreditation of graduate schools of chiropractic, whereas osteopathy has been fully subsumed under the credentialing processes of mainstream medicine.[11]

By contrast, other fields of complementary medicine are sparsely represented. There are fewer than 10,000 licensed acupuncturists in the United States, with licensure available in most states and DC. Approximately 3,000 are physician–acupuncturists, and the remainder of this category would also include a number of traditional Chinese practitioners. There are approximately 3,000 homeopaths, most of them licensed physicians. There are approximately 3,000 naturopaths, with licensure available only in a dozen states, primarily in the northwestern United States and New England and five accredited graduate schools, primarily in the northwest and southwest. Naturopaths represent the practice of an eclectic style of medicine and western herbalism, drawing from the herbal traditions of other cultures worldwide.

Perhaps some hundreds of Ayurvedic practitioners exist—many following highly individuated practices, with others ascribing to a tightly controlled Maharishi Ayur Veda school of practice. In another tradition from India, some thousands of yoga masters offer somewhat attenuated training in a variety of yoga practices, primarily designed as a meditative practice intended to influence the physical body and emotional well-being. Although there are many varieties, most practices in the United States are based on hatha yoga, which emphasizes the physical body.[19]

Energy healers now come from several organized schools of energy healing nationwide, and the practice of energy healing is widely incorporated among many members of the nursing profession in the United States through healing touch and therapeutic touch and among a number of physical therapists who may also include craniosacral therapy.[19] It is more difficult to determine the number the practitioners of Reiki and Qi Gong.

MODELS OF THERAPEUTIC INTEGRATION

To provide integrated care, state governments require that practitioners be credentialed and licensed or that existing, Western health care providers receive proper training and credentialing. Housing integrative medicine in the health care system provides credibility and legitimacy and ensures appropriate practice environments. The health care system has opportunities to make capital investments in integrated medicine facilities to provide the kind of care that is not generally available. Often the success of the integrated care clinic is based on attracting the individual practitioner's existing client base. At the same time, the individual practitioner is attracted to integrative medicine clinics by the potential for new referrals and a wider client base. Most patients come to integrative centers for the combination of CAM and allopathic medicine. An important area for expansion of services occurs when traditional health care providers refer their patients, both inpatient and outpatient, to integrated clinics.

In response to consumer demand, some managed care systems have offered access to a network of complementary care providers who have agreed to accept negotiated rates, as in other areas of health care practice. An innovative approach is to create networks of licensed holistic health providers; some plans offer an insurance rider to employers, unions, and associations for member access to services at negotiated rates. More research is needed to confirm the cost-saving potential of CAM and integrative medicine. Meanwhile, managed care systems and other insurers may do well to resist the temptation of simply adding CAM to allopathic treatment, thereby increasing health care costs.

Health care systems, hospitals, and academic medical centers offer an opportunity to develop not only the integration of appropriate complementary modalities into the continuum of care, but to develop the integration of clinical research and training with the practice of integrative medicine. A large and growing national consortium of academic medical centers (Consortium of Academic Health Centers in Integrative Medicine) has also been formed to help foster the development of integrative medical practice, research, and training, but it has been working with very limited resources.

Challenges arise with hospital policies involving integration of approved research protocols with approved practices. For example, a hospital clinic may organize to participate in a trial of an alternative infusion therapy that is approved for research. However, the costs of special staffing, equipment, and space for the research project may not be feasible unless the clinic is also approved to offer profitable infusion therapies as a service. Thus, the clinic cannot benefit over the short term to offset operating costs of research with operating revenues, and cannot benefit over the long term when the new therapy is proven to be effective if the therapy is not approved to be offered in the hospital clinic. These challenges may be addressed through adequate and realistic support for research and an integrated internal hospital policy process.

Integrated care has been taken to imply the provision of various medical modalities under the supervision of a physician. To the extent that such physician-supervised centers function as full (or even fuller)-service primary care facilities, there has been concern expressed that if primary care gatekeepers refer patients for complementary care, they may never come back. The national American WholeHealth Network, based on a successful model clinic in Chicago to provide integrated medical services under physician supervision, was unable to receive adequate referrals and had to embark on costly direct-to-consumer marketing. American WholeHealth subsequently underwent a radical shift in business strategy. Clinic managers opined that it would be necessary to receive a partial subsidy to provide the kind of care they wanted to provide, as revenues from operations under the existing health care system were inadequate to cover costs. One response to the concern about physician referrals developed by the late William Fair, Sr., a leader in integrated care, was a facility for complementary care *not* supervised by a physician. This concept, initially developed as Synergy Health opened in New York City under the name Haelth (spelled as indicated here).

Although not all physician-supervised facilities require a referral for insurance purposes, many still must rely on patient referrals from other physicians to maintain an active practice. Not all insurance plans that offer some coverage require referrals, especially not if only discounts have been negotiated.

Another important implication of integrated medicine takes the provision of complementary care beyond the primary care provider and gatekeeper to the integration of appropriate complementary medical modalities into medical specialty practice for the management of chronic diseases. The initial primary care focus of integrated medicine is being supplemented by the availability of information on integrative medicine targeted to medical specialists. Cancer care is perhaps the best example.[20]

THERAPEUTIC EFFECTIVENESS AND COST-EFFECTIVENESS

The alternative/complementary medicine research program at the NIH has increasingly emphasized clinical trials research to help create a database for evidence on the efficacy or lack of efficacy of available therapeutic modalities.[12] The health care system now has access to increasingly available, abundant, and credible information on effectiveness. In order to better understand the appropriateness and cost-effectiveness of these therapeutic modalities, it is important to expand efforts into health care utilization research. Factors such as patient motivation and satisfaction, willingness to pay for care, preference of one effective modality of care for another, and willingness to substitute care also must be studied. The development of multidisciplinary guidelines for best practices in disease management and related types of analyses that include CAM should be performed to better inform health care decision makers, whether policy makers, administrators, or consumers.

The Agency for Healthcare Research and Quality has worked within a limited budget to provide important analyses of the effectiveness and cost-effectiveness of various modalities for the management of low back pain where pharmaceuticals, surgery, spinal manual therapy,[21] acupuncture, massage, and other therapies are all present at various levels of availability, cost, and effectiveness. If improved effectiveness and cost savings are to be realized by consumers, the health system, and third-party payers, it is incumbent on integrative medicine to determine which kinds of therapeutic options can be appropriately and specifically provided to which patients in what order for cost-effective disease management. In this way the development of individualizable profiles and protocols for patients most likely to respond to various therapeutic modalities may ultimately provide a legitimate basis for increased levels of effectiveness and satisfaction at lower costs; it may also advance the provision of individualized care. These susceptibility scales or profiles may ultimately increase effectiveness and satisfaction. There is also reason to believe that individualized integrative care would lower costs.

Another aspect of cost that must be addressed today is risk management, including malpractice claims and awards and the rising costs of malpractice insurance coverage. Many practitioners claim anecdotal reports and personal experiences that integrative medical modalities have fewer and less serious side effects, reducing cause for malpractice, and that the direct relationship with practitioners and other factors reduces motivation to pursue malpractice actions. These claims need to be studied in a rigorous manner.

Side effects that are reported tend to occur through the increasingly well-known and understood potential adverse interactions of (primarily) herbal dietary supplements with regular pharmaceuticals, anesthesia, and medical procedures (see chapters 8 and 9). While responsibility for adverse interactions tends to be laid primarily at the feet of alternative modalities in the medical literature (see chapters 8 and 9), it is unlikely that biomedical products and procedures will be exempted by the legal system in considering claims and awards for damages resulting from such interactions.

MEDICAL EDUCATION

The issues considered thus far point to the clear need for enhanced and improved education at the medical school, postgraduate medical, and continuing medical education (CME) levels. CME programs are met with the challenge that current practitioners have generally had no exposure in medical school or in postgraduate medical training.

According to surveys conducted by the Center for Research in Medical Education at Thomas Jefferson University, most of today's medical students in all graduation years and among all classes want more education in integrative medicine. The proportion is increasing with each graduating year. Among classes in medical school, the proportion is relatively high in the first year (when entering students carry the culture of the general population), declines somewhat in the second and third years (as students become professionalized and generally witness little reinforcement for the teaching of integrative medicine), and rises again in the fourth year (after students have been exposed to the problems and questions of patients).[22]

The literature on integrative medicine is in the process of creation. There is considerable need for both basic science and clinical research with texts and journals reporting on both.

Much curriculum development and faculty development also remains to be done in this area. Given the potential of integrative medicine to improve health care and reduce costs, the traditional support of state and federal governments for medical education and training could be well utilized to help provide medical schools with the needed resources and incentives. In the interim, it is incumbent on providers of health care services to help stimulate appropriate CME and in-service training for health professions staff so that practitioners can be knowledgeable and helpful to their patients in seeking guidance on the use of integrative medicine.

PUBLIC POLICY ISSUES

State governments have developed a role in regulating medical practice and in supporting medical education. The federal government also maintains a unique and critical role in stimulating and supporting medical research, regulating medical products and devices, protecting the public health, and helping build health care infrastructure. All in all, government now pays more than one-third of the costs of health care in America. Policy makers at the state and federal levels should become more knowledgeable about the needs and opportunities relative to integrative medicine. The bipartisan Congressional Caucus on Complementary and Alternative Medicine and Dietary Supplements was organized for this purpose and cochaired in the Senate by Tom Harkin (D-Iowa) and Orrin Hatch (R-Utah) and in the House of Representatives by Dan Burton (R-Indiana) who also chaired the Government Reform Committee and its Subcommittee on Health and Human Rights.

It is unlikely that the current regulatory scheme governing dietary supplements (Dietary Supplement Health and Education Act of 1994, as amended 1998), which does not require premarketing proof of safety and efficacy of products sold as dietary supplements, will be significantly changed in the near future.[23] While funding for NCCAM increased each

year commensurate with the multiyear doubling of the overall NIH budget, it is critical that other federal agencies charged with programs relative
to health resources and services, primary care, health professions training,
workforce development, consumer education, health services research,
and other areas be brought to bear on the important challenge and opportunity of integrative medicine. Integrative medicine has an important
role that requires further articulation in current congressional actions on
medical liability insurance reform and the national patient safety and
quality assurance initiative. States can work together and in coordination
with the federal government to expand access to a vital complement to
traditional health care, one that has the potential to improve our health
care system. Public support together with private innovation has been the
hallmark for medical advancement in the 20th century and should continue to be the case for integrative medicine in the 21st.

CHAPTER 2

A Changing Health Care Market

Forces Shaping the Shift

BIOMEDICAL DOMINANCE

For the first half of the 20th century, health care in the United States was dominated by the biomedical model. All aspects of health care delivery, including licensing and reimbursement, reflected the authority, autonomy, and influence of the medical profession and the organizational strength of the American Medical Association (AMA). Armed with the Flexner Report, the AMA successfully warded off competition from irregulars and quacks. Stigmatized modalities went underground, suppressed but not obliterated. The 1960s ushered in a series of developments that eventually changed the face of American health care. One of these movements came to be known as complementary and alternative medicine (CAM). Consumer interest in such therapies as acupuncture and traditional Oriental medicine, herbal and nutritional care, chiropractic, massage, body-oriented psychotherapy, homeopathy, spirituality, prayer, and much more led to a movement to incorporate self-care and holistic approaches into health care. These approaches can be described as focusing on the whole person, with health viewed as depending on not only physical markers, but also emotional, mental, environmental, nutritional, and even spiritual factors. In the ensuing two decades, the use of CAM grew. Today it occupies one-third or more of consumer demand for health care services (Chapter 1).

A number of developments in the 1990s facilitated rapid growth in the use of CAM as well as interest in its healing potential. In 1991, Congress created a small Office for the Study of Unconventional Medical

Practices within the National Institutes of Health (NIH) and charged the office with investigating and providing a clearinghouse for information regarding such practices. The establishment of this office was prompted in large part by the personal experiences of Senator Tom Harkin, who had used bee pollen to relieve asthma, and Representative Berkeley Bedell, who had used a non-FDA-approved substance to help treat prostate cancer. The office's mandate and very existence were controversial at inception and have continued to generate controversy. Nevertheless, Congress has repeatedly approved renewed and increased funding. The office, which became the National Center for Complementary and Alternative Medicine (NCCAM) in 1998, is helping to build a scientific foundation for understanding the safety and efficacy of specific CAM therapies. The research it funds and the findings, which are now regularly published in mainstream medical journals, as well as in medical literature that has evolved to support publication specifically devoted to the growing number of CAM articles, are having a direct and positive impact on attitudes toward CAM within conventional medicine.

In addition to the research, physicians' attitudes toward CAM have been influenced by their patients' growing use, as well as by surveys revealing that patients hesitate to inform doctors about their use of CAM.[24] When patients do want to discuss CAM with their physicians, it is often to ask for advice; however, physicians on the whole have not been sufficiently well informed to comply. Spurred by these developments as well as their own interests, physicians are participating in the many continuing medical education courses on CAM offered by major medical schools across the country. Some physicians are even becoming CAM practitioners themselves. At the same time, almost 60% of U.S. medical schools are offering courses on CAM to meet the demand of medical students.

Other health care providers, most importantly hospitals, are also taking heed of the flow of patients to CAM practitioners. A 2000–2001 survey of 5,810 hospitals by the American Hospital Association reported that 15% of the respondents offered CAM therapies.[25] Those offered most frequently (combining inpatient and outpatient services) were pastoral care, massage therapy, relaxation treatment, guided imagery, and therapeutic nutrition. Services less likely to be offered were naturopathy, homeopathy, chiropractic, medical symptom reduction, and reflexology. The survey concluded that 49% of respondents viewed patient demand as the primary motivation for offering these services, while another 24% stated that offering them reflected their organizational mission.

Although some CAM services continue to be provided on an ad hoc basis, within the last several years a growing number of hospitals have begun to institutionalize their provision through the establishment of integrative health care centers (IHCs). IHCs represent the latest evolutionary stage in the growth of CAM, reflecting not only a linguistic innovation but also a revolutionary development in the practice of health care. Integration is taking CAM beyond simple mainstreaming by actively coordinating its modalities with those of conventional medicine. Although the promise of integrative health care is enormous, the task of establishing IHCs has not been altogether smooth. There are few guidelines or models for those venturing into this novel realm of health care. A 2005 survey studied 39 randomly selected academic medical centers integrating complementary and alternative medical (CAM) services into conventional care.[26] The study found that 23 offered CAM services—usually acupuncture, massage, dietary supplements, mind–body therapies, and music therapy. A 2004 survey of 33 academic health centers revealed that 95% of academic centers surveyed provide some CAM clinical care. Acupuncture and massage were most common, with naturopathy and homeopathy least common.[27]

But CAM has entered many other medical settings as well, even care settings that might have been perceived as conservative or resistant to CAM therapies, such as the military. For example, a survey published in the May 2004 issue of *Military Medicine* found that military families are among those that routinely use CAM therapies, including massage therapy, nutritional food supplements, herbal supplements, exercise therapy, chiropractic, music therapy, relaxation therapy, aromatherapy, meditation, magnet therapy, biofeedback, acupuncture, Tai Chi, yoga, naturopathy, homeopathy, Qi Gong, and hypnotherapy. CAM therapies were used to treat conditions such as lower back pain, stress, weight loss, neck pain, headaches, knee pain, upper back pain, shoulder pain, anxiety, depression, migraines, colds, hip pain, wrist pain, stomach pain, chronic fatigue syndrome, pelvic pain, sinus pain, viral conditions, and fibromyalgia and for health prevention (preventive medicine).[28]

This same study echoed findings of a government survey released in May 2004 that some 36% of U.S. adults aged 18 years and over use some form of CAM.[29] This survey, administered to more than 31,000 representative U.S. adults, was conducted as part of the Centers for Disease Control and Prevention's (CDC) 2002 National Health Interview Survey (NHIS). Developed by NCCAM and the CDC's National Center for Health Statistics (NCHS), the survey included questions on 27 types of CAM therapies commonly used in the United States.

Doubtless the growing interest in integrative medicine is also fueled by, and also has parallels to, other social movements such as environmentalism and awareness of so-called green alternatives to present energy sources.[30] In any event, as indicated by the *Report on Complementary and Alternative Medicine* published in 2005 by the Institute of Medicine, National Academy of Sciences: "The data presented indicate that hospitals, managed care organizations, and conventional practitioners have incorporated some CAM therapies into the provision of health care services."[31]

SIGNIFICANT LEGAL AND REGULATORY DEVELOPMENTS

The law governing CAM practitioners and therapies grows out of, and overlaps with, several different areas of law governing conventional care, for example, licensing, malpractice liability, and food and drug law.[32] A growing number of statutes and cases are beginning to address legal issues specific to CAM, such as licensing of CAM practitioners (e.g., acupuncturists and massage therapists); professional discipline for conventional providers who use CAM therapies without adequate education, training, or skill; potential malpractice liability of providers and health care organizations incorporating CAM therapies; application of relevant food and drug law; and third-party reimbursement for CAM therapies.[33] Yet, to date few authors have addressed the legal and regulatory implications of including CAM therapies and providers in conventional health care settings or offered specific guidance to institutions seeking to include such therapies and providers.

Similarly, much of the medical literature to date has presented debates for or against the very notion of CAM therapies and described objections to allowing consumers access to them, absent general medical acceptance.[34] But little attention has been paid to the criteria hospitals should use to allow (or disallow) specific providers and therapies. Because of this lack of guidance, one hospital reported simply giving up trying to craft an institutional policy to handle patient interest in dietary supplements.[35] The lapse reflected the institution's inability to reach consensus and the imprecision of current standards regarding quality assurance for dietary supplements rather than any definitive evidence of lack of safety or efficacy for any given product or products. We expect that this is not an isolated experience.

Despite the battles around the evidence base (or lack thereof) for one or more CAM therapies and the inattention to creating meaningful guidelines, hospitals increasingly are beginning to provide patients with various modalities, ranging from chiropractic to massage therapy to mind–body techniques. Simultaneously, a number of CAM therapies are becoming generally accepted or recognized to have demonstrated safety and efficacy. On the regulatory front, new statutes are changing the way unlicensed providers are regulated in some states.[36] There has also been a White House Commission on Complementary and Alternative Medicine

Policy, whose final report to the U.S. President recommended mechanisms to increase nationwide consumer access to CAM therapies and the creation of a federal office to oversee federal implementation of certain recommendations.[37] Mainstream medicine has joined in credible efforts to report on CAM research, clinical practice, and policy, with, as noted, a Report on Complementary and Alternative Medicine by the Institute of Medicine in 2005.

In succeeding chapters, we examine some of the legal and regulatory issues for institutional policy as practitioners, clinics, hospitals, and other health care organizations (including managed care groups) work to understand liability and other legal implications of incorporating CAM therapies and practitioners into conventional medical settings. We show how novel issues involving credentialing, malpractice liability, and risk management and policies involving dietary supplements can be creatively addressed if health care institutions are to respond to patient interest in CAM in ways that provide therapeutic benefit yet satisfy liability concerns. We also focus on risk management quandaries faced by institutions attempting integration of evidence-based CAM therapies and on reports of success or failure with specific credentialing, liability management, and dietary supplements policies to date.

By presenting strategies and model policies used to implement clinical models of integrative care, we help health care institutions break out of the stagnation of "don't ask, and don't tell."[38] These models, in turn, will propel the implementation of health care practices involving CAM therapies that are clinically appropriate, ethically responsible, and legally defensible in conventional medical settings.

UNDERSTANDING AND DEFINING CAM

The term *alternative medicine* has elicited considerable misunderstanding. It is a double misnomer, purporting to describe health care services that may not necessarily be either "alternative" to medicine or "medical." Derived not from any consensus within the medical community, but from political, legislative, and sociological developments, changes in terminology have reflected changes in these broader movements (chapter 1).

Consider the original name of the Office for the Study of Unconventional Medical Practices. The term *unconventional* suggests a history of antipathy by biomedicine toward its economic competitors and rivals, echoed in the prevailing political winds and lack of medical acceptability for the referent therapies. The debate goes back to the late 18th and 19th centuries. Harvard Medical School's Oliver Wendell Holmes called homeopathy a "mingled mass of perverse ingenuity, of tinsel erudition, of imbecile credulity, and of artful misrepresentation," while the "irregular" practitioners responded with epithets and "witch-hunted any of their own who might adopt 'enemy' therapeutics and beliefs."[39] At an address to the Massachusetts Medical Society (publisher of the *New England Journal of Medicine*) in 1860 Holmes also stated, "if the entire material media as currently practiced could be thrown to the bottom of the sea, it would be all the better for mankind and all the worse for the fishes."

The modern term *unconventional* described holistic healing practices from the vantage of conventional physicians, much in the way that the term *unorthodox therapies* was being juxtaposed against those therapies accepted by medical orthodoxy. Holistic therapies lived in the world of *"un's* and *non's"*—they were *unconventional, unorthodox, unproven,* and *nonbiomedical.* They were known to the medical establishment primarily by what they were not.

With burgeoning consumer demand in the 1980s, labels began to shift and the term *alternative medicine* was introduced. As a parallel development within the legal and medical communities, there was growing recognition of the importance of consumer autonomy through the doctrine of informed consent and growing recognition of the fact that medical technology has limits and may dehumanize the patient. In 1993, a landmark article published in the *New England Journal of Medicine* revealed that at least one in three Americans was using these therapies.[40] The article defined *alternative medical practices* to include therapies not commonly used in U.S. hospitals or taught in U.S. medical schools.

As the term *alternative medicine* continued to gain political currency, the Office at the NIH was renamed the Office of Alternative Medicine (OAM). The term *alternative*, though, again had political connotations. It still defined therapies within its rubric in contradistinction to biomedicine; indeed, the therapies were conspicuously absent from most of biomedical education and practice. Although useful as a starting point for understanding certain modalities, the definition increasingly became outdated. By the mid-1990s alternative therapies were being incorporated into the curriculum of major medical schools—albeit largely as upper-level, elective courses—and slowly began filtering into departments in major U.S. hospitals.

In the United Kingdom and Europe, the term *complementary medicine* was entering the mainstream nomenclature as a more neutral way to describe therapies that were sometimes used instead of biomedical care but more frequently used to complement biomedical therapies (for example, in-hospital massage for stress reduction and relief from depression; acupuncture to alleviate nausea following chemotherapy). Heeding public demand and supported by a British Medical Association report,[41] the National Health Service began in the 1990s to cover general practitioner referrals to homeopaths and acupuncturists. Reflecting a diffusion of terminology, the notion of "complementary and alternative medical" therapies began to gain ground in many academic and government circles in the United States as a way to describe the phenomenon and create more credibility than the earlier notion of alternative medicine.

Accordingly, by 1998, after a dedicated effort by proponents of CAM therapies, the NIH office was elevated to a national center. Unlike the OAM, its predecessor, the NCCAM was given its own grant-making authority and capability and a budget that had grown exponentially since the initial $2 million annual fund. Today, NCCAM has a robust research program for CAM therapies. The Center's Web site officially defines CAM as, "a group of diverse medical and health care systems, practices, and products that are not presently considered to be part of conventional medicine."[42] But this definition also suffers from ambiguity, since not all CAM therapies are medical, and many CAM therapies can be incorporated into conventional medicine once generally accepted within the medical community.

A different but related way to view CAM is as "a broad domain of healing resources that accompanies all health care systems, modalities and practices, and their accompanying theories and beliefs other than those intrinsic to the politically dominant health care of a particular society or culture within a given period."[43] While perhaps true historically, given biomedical dominance in health care, this definition today is still problematic, because the contours of which group or subgroup is "politically dominant" may shift from time to time or in a given context. It may be more accurate to say that CAM includes a broad range of modalities that historically had fallen outside of conventional care—such as chiropractic, naturopathy, massage therapy, acupuncture and traditional Oriental medicine, nutritional and herbal medicine, folk medicine, spirituality in medicine, and mind–body therapies—but that increasingly are part of a web of professional care and self-care networks.

To complicate matters, CAM therapies may be provided by medical doctors and other allied health providers (e.g., physicians counseling patients regarding their use or avoidance of herbs; nurses offering massage), or by specially trained CAM practitioners (e.g., acupuncture offered by a licensed practitioner of traditional Oriental medicine). In addition, therapies may be offered by conventional providers—particularly in the area of mind–body medicine—that could be considered either biomedical or within the CAM domain (e.g., psychologists offering guided imagery and visualization). Further, the reasons for defining individual modalities as "CAM therapies" are not solely either medical or legal. Rather, reasons include "political, social, or conceptual" rationales,[44] such as the fact that the amount of data or type of data is considered insufficient or otherwise inadequate (e.g., herbalism, megavitamin therapy); the amount of research funding, infrastructure, and capacity for investigating the practice is low (e.g., massage, chiropractic); the practice is not reimbursed by insurance companies and third-party payers; the practice is not readily used for feasibility, acceptability, or other reasons (e.g., clinical ecology, complex lifestyle programs); or the practice is not regulated or licensed in most states (e.g., naturopathy). Defining CAM and its use, appropriateness, and relation to regulatory and hospital policy is a multifaceted and complex problem.

Beyond wrangling over the proper place of CAM therapies in conventional care—or debates around the appropriateness of pluralism in health care or in the scientific methodology used to decide safety and effectiveness of nonbiomedical modalities—consumer demand for and utilization of these therapies continues to increase. A 1998 follow-up to the 1993 study found a 47% increase in total visits to CAM practitioners, from 427 million in 1990 to 629 million in 1997, with total 1997 out-of-pocket expenditures relating to CAM therapies estimated at 27 billion dollars.[45] The study suggested that use of complementary and alternative medicine is likely to continue to increase, particularly as insurance reimbursement for these therapies grows. As suggested, more recent data have shown that the number of CAM users is indeed increasing.

In short, terms such as *alternative* and even *complementary* no longer accurately describe the market for these health care services, though CAM is generally used as consensus nomenclature. Today, physicians are increasingly recognizing that to guide patients in their use of CAM therapies, they must be knowledgeable about such therapies.

TOWARD INTEGRATIVE HEALTH CARE

As health care organizations begin to include CAM therapies within the conventional medical setting or refer patients to CAM practitioners affiliated with a hospital or a provider network, the terms *integrative medicine* or *integrative health care* have come to define the effort to offer biomedical and CAM therapies within a conventional health care delivery system. Once again, nomenclature defines consciousness and policy, and several definitions are emerging within the medical community. NCCAM, for example, presently defines integrative medicine as health care that "combines mainstream medical therapies and CAM therapies for which there is some high-quality scientific evidence of safety and effectiveness."[46] By way of comparison, within the medical literature a relatively new proposed definition attempts to distinguish the emerging notion of integrative health care from the 5- to 10-year-old definition of CAM therapies:

Importantly, in one definition, *integrative care* is not synonymous with *complementary and alternative medicine* (CAM). It has a far larger meaning and mission in that it calls for restoration of the focus of medicine on health and healing and emphasizes the centrality of the patient–physician relationship.[47]

This definition emphasizes the therapeutic relationship rather than the particular therapy:

> In addition to providing the best conventional care, integrative medicine focuses on preventative maintenance of health by paying attention to all relative components of lifestyle, including diet, exercise, stress management, and emotional well-being. It insists on patients being active participants in their health care as well as on physicians viewing patients as whole persons—minds, community members, and spiritual beings, as well as physical bodies.[48]

This definition incorporates holistic notions of CAM therapies into the medical world. Further, although it emphasizes changes within the medical profession, it does not suggest a decline in biomedical dominance. Greater parity may evolve between medical and other providers and systems of knowledge about human health and disease. But it is not imminent.[49] Accordingly, the definition simply "asks physicians to serve as guides, role models, and mentors, as well as dispensers of therapeutic aids."[50]

Yet another potential definition for integrative health care describes a system of medicine that seeks to provide *safe, effective, and appropriate* care in the best interest of the patient as it integrates complementary and alternative medicine with conventional care.[51] Such a definition of integration includes perspectives such as concern for patient autonomy and consumer choice, as well as evidence-based medical decision making. This notion of integration implies "building on existing models, discarding what is conclusively shown to be dangerous and ineffective, yet evolving new ideas based on emerging information and perception."[52]

ANCHORING AN IDEAL

Consensus definitions affect institutional as well as regulatory policy, as we noted earlier. Without consensus, integrative health care remains an ideal without an anchor. By opening clinical centers specifically devoted to offering patients some combination of CAM and biomedical therapies within the conventional medical setting, many hospitals are presently pioneering models of integrative care. They are doing so without the benefit of reproducible models, based on generally accepted legal, ethical, and clinical parameters for such care. This leaves them at risk of internal criticism and dissolution, as well as of threats to financial viability and unresolved issues of potential liability.

In part, the reality of such risk results from the novelty of integrative health care: Insufficient research has been done to determine the best clinical pathway for treatment of a specific condition in a way that most efficiently uses both biomedical and CAM practitioners. For example, should a patient with tennis elbow see a chiropractor first and then an acupuncturist, followed by a neurologist, or the reverse? Should a medical doctor be consulted for a patient evaluation before the patient sees any CAM practitioner, or does this arrangement leave biomedicine in the dominant position, as gatekeeper to other services? These kinds of questions combine issues of clinical judgment, research evidence, legal and liability considerations, and political, cultural, and philosophical issues about the role of medicine in an "integrated" health care system that includes a variety of providers historically shunned by biomedicine.

In addition, a number of sociological, economic, political, and ethical factors have precluded the creation of definitive models for successful integration. Professional and institutional biases against certain CAM therapies and practitioners can create barriers to true integration. For example, should chiropractors be made part of the medical staff—and is this feasible in most hospitals, given the historical antipathy by medical doctors toward the chiropractic profession?[53] Do massage therapists and energy healers have a role to play with the dying patient, given existing debates about compassionate use of pain medication and other care at the end of life?[54] Is it appropriate for physicians to allow patients under their care to continue taking dietary supplements, where the evidence concerning safety and efficacy is less than reassuring?[55]

Such questions set the terms for ongoing institutional and regulatory debates. While current scholarly material offers no definitive answers, institutional experiences are forging new models and boundaries. Thus, although some such questions initially depend on interpretations of state law (for example, malpractice rules, including rules governing informed consent; licensing laws for nonmedical, CAM practitioners and the scope of practice boundaries these laws authorize for such providers), potential solutions also turn on local politics, preferences, and predilections.

For these reasons, resolving some of the present conundrums of integrative care is not only theoretical and rhetorical, but also requires data from the actual experiences of institutions attempting to implement such care in conventional medical settings. Our narrative case studies serve this purpose. (In a few of these case studies we combine stories from multiple institutions where similar narratives contribute to elaboration of the same theme.)

ABOUT INTEGRATIVE MEDICINE CENTERS

We designed a study to evaluate the major legal and social challenges hospitals are facing in implementing integrative health care as well as successful strategies used to overcome them. We focused on the following four areas:

1. *Credentialing standards* and procedures for licensed CAM practitioners (e.g., chiropractors, acupuncturists, and massage therapists) to serve as members of the clinical team within an integrative health care setting.
2. *Policies and procedures to minimize malpractice risk* exposure in integrative health care practices.
3. *Guidelines regarding pharmacy and therapeutics* committee practices as they relate to the use or avoidance of herbal products and other dietary supplements for outpatients and inpatients.
4. *Institutional, political, and social support structures* needed to develop integrative health care centers; the role of market forces in shaping programs in the centers; and the role of scientific and medical knowledge in guiding responsible delivery of integrative health care.[56]

See Appendix A for a list of interview questions we asked.

We drew our interview sample from the top 50 research medical schools and the top 50 primary medical schools, as rated by *U. S. News and World Report*.[57] Of this total of 56 schools (not all appeared on both lists), 27 have active or newly established integrative health care centers with clinical programs. We interviewed key personnel at 23 of these centers; four did not respond to our second request for an interview. Included in this sample are several members of the Consortium of Academic Health Centers for Integrative Medicine, a group of major academic medical centers that have explicit administrative support (and seed funding) to explore common research and educational issues in integrative care.[58] Because of their prominence within medicine and/or the prestige and size of the affiliated institution, some of the centers and personnel interviewed generally could be considered leaders or pioneers in the field of integrative health care. Many represent a second wave of academic entrepreneurs whose involvement came after it was demonstrated by others that it was "safe to go into the water." Also included in the sample are a number of centers devoted to oncology (cancer care). The use of integrative medicine in cancer care is perhaps the most dramatic example of integration invoking the issues presented in this book.[20] See Appendix B for a list of centers whose directors gave consent to be listed.

We received Institutional Review Board approval from Beth Israel Deaconess Medical Center and Harvard Medical School, with the understanding that consent would be given by participation and verbal agreement. We also gave assurances of confidentiality—namely, that the identities of individual centers and center personnel would be masked, and any identifying information unique to particular individuals or institutions redacted from the quotations.

We conducted 15-minute to 1-hour face-to-face and telephone interviews with key personnel in the selected, integrative health care centers regarding their major challenges and the strategies they used to overcome obstacles in the preceding four areas. Among the personnel we interviewed were (1) the center administrator or executive director (if differing from category 3, following); (2) legal counsel affiliated with the center or larger hospital; (3) medical or clinical director for the center; (4) representative sample of conventional and CAM practitioners (e.g., nurse, physical therapist, psychologist, acupuncturist, massage therapist, chiropractor); and (5) pharmacist affiliated with the center or larger hospital.

Interviews were semistructured, aiming to elicit subjective impressions of the chief legal, regulatory, and internal political challenges and strategies used to surmount obstacles in the attempt to gain acceptance and authorization for integrative care within the health care institution. Between July 2002 and March 2004 we conducted more than 70 interviews with key personnel in the integrative health care centers selected.

The institutions we studied were diverse in size, location, and focus, included all major geographic sections of the country, and ranged from large medical centers with multiple health care schools and affiliated teaching hospitals to smaller centers with a single professional school (medicine) and teaching hospital. Our focus was the integrative health care centers themselves; we did not study isolated CAM practitioners either elsewhere within or outside the institution (for example, the acupuncturist affiliated on a full- or part-time basis with a hospital's pain unit or the chiropractor outside the hospital to whom a surgeon might from time to time make a referral).

A note on terminology: Integrative health care centers can have one or more of three different programs—clinical, research, or education. Some centers are confined to only one of these programs. Our focus in this book is on the clinical component of the centers, and we emphasized in our selection only those centers that have a clinical program. When we wish to specify the clinical unit or function, we use the term *clinic*. Otherwise, we use the term *center*. In some academic settings, the term *center* has both administrative and political connotations that circumscribe its use. Even though some of the IHCs in our study may not refer to themselves as centers, we use the term here.

We acknowledge two major limitations in our research process. First, it is difficult, if not impossible, to create a study sample that can be generalized, simply because the field of integrative health care is so new in medicine and because models of integration differ at each institution. For example, the first six academic medical centers sampled in our study provide enormous diversity. One institution was the first clinical site of an early, prominent academic medical center, but since has become a nonprofit, community hospital, with its own free-standing medical, psychiatry, and other departments. Another institution is a mind–body clinic that operates in conjunction with a community health system, and whose ownership has been transferred from a university to the community health system, and may be transferred back (or, alternatively, the clinic may close). A third institution was located within an academic medical center, then closed as a result of financial pressures, and later reopened as an independent, for-profit clinic that has a teaching relationship with the medical center.

Even across similar institutions, each integrative health care center has a particular view of what constitutes an integrative care team. Some centers, for example, include acupuncturists but not massage therapists; others, the reverse. Some have a psychiatrist as the mind–body provider offering such therapies as hypnosis and biofeedback, whereas others rely on a psychologist or a master of social work; some have nurses providing therapies such as Reiki, while others allow their massage therapists to offer energy therapies with bodywork. One has a physician-homeopath plus a chiropractor.

A second limitation involves the difficulty in standardizing interviews across institutions, in terms of length, specificity of topics covered, and consistency of personnel. Interviewees had different time constraints. Questions followed the flow of conversation and the thread of local conditions. Gaining access to key personnel such as legal counsel was difficult; some centers, because of their delicate relationships with hospital administration and general distrust of lawyers, expressed fear of providing such a contact. Many centers did not have access to affiliated pharmacists; others had few providers from whom to solicit interviews.

Despite these limitations, some common themes and strategies emerged. Center leaders and staff are working creatively to expand outreach and referral bases across academic medical departments, achieve financial sustainability, incorporate research programs, translate research findings into clinical care, and establish permanence within their home institutions. Integrative medicine is a relatively new phenomenon in U.S. health care, but its contours already are offering new models and possibilities for care across clinical disciplines.

CHAPTER 3

Assessing the Landscape

Key Legal and Institutional Forces

LEGAL ISSUES GOVERNING INDIVIDUAL PROVIDERS

Legal rules governing CAM and integrative care by health care professionals and institutions are extensive. There are five major categories: (1) licensure, (2) scope of practice, (3) professional discipline, (4) malpractice, and (5) fraud.[59] These arenas of law work together as complex levers of limitations on potential abuse of practice authority in a variety of situations. They apply across the board to physicians and nonphysicians (both conventional, such as nurses and physical therapists, and CAM providers, such as chiropractors and acupuncturists). Most of these rules apply to individual providers of CAM therapies, though, as we discuss, there also may be implications for institutions.

Medical Licensure

Medical licensure is one of the earliest forms of regulation recognizing professional delivery of health care services and subjecting the conduct of health care professionals to statutory proscriptions.[60] Medical licensure originated in the colony of New York in 1760 as a means to prevent "ignorant and unskillful persons" from "endangering the lives and limbs of their patients, and many poor and ignorant persons, who have been persuaded to become their patients."[61] The statutory definition of practicing medicine varies by state, but typically includes (1) diagnosing, preventing, treating, and curing disease; (2) holding oneself out to the public as able to perform the preceding activities; (3) intending to receive a gift, fee, or compensation for the preceding activities; (4) attaching such titles as MD to one's name; (5) maintaining an office for reception, examination, and treatment; (6) performing surgery; and (7) using, administering, or prescribing drugs or medicinal preparations.[62]

By requiring a license to practice "medicine" and defining the practice of medicine in its broadest sense, any act constituting "diagnosis" or "treatment" for any disease or ailment—medical licensing laws, as interpreted by courts, resulted in convictions of chiropractors, naturopaths, massage therapists, hypnotists, nutritional counselors, and spiritual healers for unlicensed medical practice.[63] Thus, although they were initially weakly enforced, by the late 19th century, medical licensing laws had become a powerful tool for enforcing dominant medical paradigms.[64] Medical licensure had evolved from the attempt to control lay practitioners of the healing arts into the consolidation of a medical establishment, with extensive political and economic control[65] and the ability to condemn anyone who opposed dominant medical perspectives as "an 'enemy of physic and all learning.' "[66]

Although medical licensure has been variously criticized as self-serving, ineffective, and tending to incite litigation over practice boundaries,[67] its ostensible purpose—to protect the public from unscrupulous and untrained providers—arguably deters those who practice medicine under the statutory definitions from delivering health care services that could injure the public. Medical licensure thus serves the regulatory goal of fraud control.[68]

Courts have followed legislatures in conceptualizing the practice of medicine broadly, so as to include many different kinds of practitioners and practices within the proscription against practicing medicine without a license.[69] This interpretation has resulted in litigation involving allied health providers, such as psychologists, physician assistants, and nurse practitioners, as well as osteopaths, midwives, and other providers of therapies outside conventional medicine (including lay practitioners of spiritual healing).

Because medical licensing laws have resulted in convictions of spiritual healers and others for unlicensed practice of medicine, grassroots movements have grown in a number of states, seeking to free such providers from the threat of prosecution for unlicensed medical practice. For example, at least four states—California, Idaho, Minnesota, and Rhode Island—have enacted legislation permitting (with specified limitations) practice of health care by persons who are not licensed by the state.

California's legislation provides that a person is not in violation of specified provisions of the Medical Practice Act that prohibit the practice of medicine without being licensed as a physician, as long as the person does not engage in specified acts and also makes specified disclosures to each client, for which the client must acknowledge receipt in writing.[70]

Similarly, Rhode Island defines "unlicensed health care practices" as

> the broad domain of unlicensed healing methods and treatments, including, but not limited to: (i) acupressure; (ii) Alexander technique; (iii) aroma therapy; (iv) ayurveda; (v) cranial sacral therapy; (vi) crystal therapy; (vii) detoxification practices and therapies; (viii) energetic healing; (ix) rolfing; (x) Gerson therapy and colostrum therapy; (xi) therapeutic touch; (xii) herbology or herbalism; (xiii) polarity therapy; (xiv) homeopathy; (xv) nondiagnostic iridology; (xvi) body work; (xvii) reiki; (xviii) mind-body healing practices; (ixx) naturopathy; and (xx) Qi Gong energy healing.[71]

The legislation provides that subject to certain restrictions, persons in Rhode Island "are authorized to practice as unlicensed health care practitioners and receive remuneration for their services."[72] Restrictions include a posting that the state has not adopted any educational and training standards for unlicensed health care practitioners.[73]

The registration requirements provided by such laws, aimed in large part to protect such providers from unlicensed medical practice, may still leave them vulnerable to claims of exceeding competence and thereby crossing the line into unlicensed medical practice, if courts continue the historical tendency to interpret medical licensing statutes and the concepts of "diagnosis" and "treatment" broadly.[74] Further, such laws allow providers to be prosecuted if they commit fraudulent acts,[75] or are found to be engaging in contact that "may be reasonably interpreted by a client as . . . engaging in sexual exploitation,"[76] or are shown unable "to engage in unlicensed health care practices with reasonable safety to . . . clients."[77] Providers also are prohibited from offering a *medical diagnosis*, although that term, while it is more specific than simply *diagnosis*, typically is not given further definition.

As an example of pertinent prohibitions, California's legislation allows prosecution if the unlicensed provider (1) conducts surgery or any other procedure that punctures the skin or harmfully invades the body on another person; (2) administers or prescribes X-ray radiation to another person; (3) prescribes or administers legend drugs or controlled substances to another person; (4) recommends the discontinuance of legend drugs or controlled substances prescribed by an appropriately licensed practitioner; (5) willfully diagnoses and treats a physical or mental condition of any person under circumstances or conditions that cause or create a risk of great bodily harm, serious physical or mental illness, or death . . . ; (8) holds out, states, indicates, advertises, or implies to a client or prospective client that he or she is a physician, a surgeon, or a physician and surgeon.[78]

Scope of Practice Rules

Scope of practice rules spell out the health care services that licensed non-physicians (as opposed to physicians or laypersons) are authorized to provide pursuant to their own licensing statutes. Such services typically are defined more narrowly than the broad authority granted to physicians to diagnose and treat disease.[79] For example, in the allied health professions, licensure to practice psychology or physical therapy does not authorize the licensee to diagnose and treat in the medical sense.

As an example relevant to the limits of healing by nonphysician CAM practitioners, licensed chiropractors typically are authorized to use spinal manipulation and adjustment to readjust the flow of "nerve energy" in their patients; licensed acupuncturists, to use techniques of traditional Oriental medicine to help adjust the "flow and balance of energy in the body"; and licensed massage therapists to use "rubbing, stroking, kneading, or tapping" the muscles to promote relaxation and affect well-being.[80]

None of these providers are authorized to diagnose and treat disease in the medical sense. For this reason, the licensing statutes delineating scope of practice provisions for nonphysicians frequently include an express prohibition against the unlicensed practice of medicine.[81] Indeed, such providers have a duty to refer the patient to a physician whenever the patient's condition exceeds the scope of their training, education, and competence; and violation of the duty can lead to malpractice liability.[82]

Despite these statutory attempts to draw distinctions, the line between authorized practice of a nonmedical profession (e.g., chiropractic) and unauthorized medical practice can be difficult to draw. For example, chiropractors who have offered nutritional advice have been prosecuted for practicing medicine unlawfully, despite the argument that nutritional care is part of chiropractic education and training.[83] Courts have tended to interpret scope of practice narrowly, corresponding with interpreting the practice of medicine broadly and inclusively.[84]

In addition to the rationale of preserving public health, safety, and welfare, one reason for this blurring of lines is that any distinction between a holistic notion of wellness care (adopted by many CAM practitioners) and the actual diagnosis and treatment of a disease is difficult to conceptualize. The difficulty increases when the latter terms are taken in their broadest sense to incorporate any and all attempts to help patients heal.[85] In either case, many modalities such as nutritional care occupy the borderline between the two poles of "wellness care" and "disease care."[86] A further problem is that scope of practice rules "reflect the notion that the enterprise of healing can be carved into neatly severable and licensable blocks," whereas many CAM practices aim to be holistic—to address the whole person and not simply an afflicted body part.[87]

Professional Discipline

Licensing statutes for health care professionals (both physicians and non-physicians) typically include a set of provisions specifying under what circumstances the licensed professional may be disciplined, with sanctions ranging from fines to loss of licensure. Unprofessional conduct (also known as professional misconduct) that provides a basis for such discipline typically includes such acts as obtaining the license fraudulently, practicing the profession fraudulently, practicing with gross incompetence or gross negligence, practicing while impaired by drugs or alcohol, permitting or aiding an unlicensed person to practice unlawfully, or failing to comply with relevant rules and regulations.[88]

Notably, in recent years a number of states have enacted statutes protecting health care providers—particularly physicians—from professional discipline based on therapeutic recommendations involving CAM therapies. For example, Alaska's statute, enacted in 1990, states that the medical board "may not base a finding of professional incompetence solely on the basis that a licensee's practice is unconventional or experimental in the absence of demonstrable physical harm to a patient."[89] Similarly, Colorado's statute provides: "The board shall not take disciplinary action against a [physician] solely on the grounds that such a [physician] practices alternative medicine."[90] The language contained in these statutes varies by state.[91] In most states, it remains to be seen whether such language would, in fact, protect providers incorporating controversial therapies.[92]

New guidelines by the Federation of State Medical Boards concerning physician use of CAM therapies provide that in considering professional discipline, the medical board should evaluate whether the physician is using a treatment that is

- effective and safe (having adequate scientific evidence of efficacy or safety or greater safety than other established treatment models for the same condition);
- effective, but with some real or potential danger (having evidence of efficacy but also of adverse side effects);
- inadequately studied, but safe (having insufficient evidence of clinical efficacy but reasonable evidence to suggest relative safety);
- ineffective and dangerous (proved to be ineffective or unsafe through controlled trials or documented evidence or as measured by a risk/benefit assessment).

In one sense, these categories leave much ambiguity: For example, they do not specify how and when specific judgments about levels of evidence in the gray zones are likely to trigger disciplinary action. In addition, these are only suggested guidelines, offering language that individual state medical boards are free to adopt, disregard, or look to in conjunction with existing law for a framework for handling disciplinary cases involving use of CAM therapies. The guidelines contain a wealth of details that the Federation would like physicians to follow, but this is only theoretical until a particular state legislative or regulatory body (e.g., medical board) incorporates relevant language into its regulatory framework.

Notably, the Federation guidelines have had influence in such far-flung jurisdictions as the United Arab Emirates, where the Ministry of Health has established a Complementary and Alternative Medicine Section,[93] and has enacted regulations concerning CAM practices within the seven emirates,[94] modeling these rules after sources including the Federation guidelines. It is difficult to envision how these guidelines may be applied in another culture.

And even within the United States, it is difficult to track disciplinary cases, as they rarely result in published judicial opinions and are often resolved with an agreement between the practitioner and the medical board, in which the board softens its disciplinary recommendation and the practitioner agrees to make practice changes urged by the board. For example, a physician who has used a controversial CAM therapy whose efficacy (but not safety) is questioned may not necessarily have to lose his or her license, but might be asked to discontinue the practice, or to utilize a stronger and cleared informed consent process. It is unclear whether the Federation guidelines merely offer "illusory progress" to physicians seeking to judiciously integrate CAM therapies.[95] More research is necessary to understand how medical boards are currently viewing such disciplinary cases in light of the Federation guidelines or equivalent state regulations.

Malpractice

Malpractice liability rules protect patients against negligence by health care providers. Negligent practice is defined as practicing below the standard of care, resulting in injury to the patient.

Including CAM therapies does not necessarily mean that the physician has provided substandard care. Unfortunately, however, some courts may be tempted to make this equation. For example, the court in *Charell v. Gonzales* articulated the proposition that a physician's inclusion of CAM therapies conceivably could itself be negligent, given the current definition of CAM therapies as health care modalities not generally accepted by biomedicine.[96] Given this approach, the danger of identifying provision of CAM therapies with malpractice may increase with use of a therapy such as energy healing, which has an unknown mechanism.

In *Charell*, the expert witness for the plaintiff helped persuade the jury that the defendant physician's use of a nutritional protocol was "bogus" and "of no value."[97] *Charell* is not the wisest precedent for other judges to follow, and it will be important for courts to apply the elements of malpractice rather than simply conclude malpractice from the fact that a CAM therapy that is not generally accepted within the medical profession was used.

Several defenses to medical malpractice might be available to the provider who uses a CAM therapy. These defenses might apply even if the therapy has not been adopted as part of the standard of care within the jurisdiction. The defenses include the "respectable minority" defense—the idea that a significant segment within the profession accepts the modality—and assumption of risk, the notion that the patient knowingly, voluntarily, and intelligently assumed a risk of injury from the chosen therapy.[98] The respectable minority defense, however, is especially complicated in regard to use of CAM therapies, because it may be difficult to determine what constitutes the requisite quantity of providers and what level of evidence of safety or efficacy would make them sufficiently "respectable" to trigger the defense. Similarly, the assumption of risk defense does not allow providers to act negligently; in other words, there are some risks that courts will not allow patients to assume. The defense triggers a circular argument as to what is, in fact, negligent.

A second theory supporting malpractice liability is the failure to provide adequate informed consent (see chapter 7). To date, no patient has successfully argued that a provider's failure to disclose the possibility of using a CAM therapy, instead of a biomedical therapy, caused injury and constituted malpractice. However, at least one court has observed that such an argument would succeed if the therapy in question had a sufficient level of professional acceptance.[99]

One problem with malpractice law is that frequently, the most egregious cases are the ones that come to light through published judicial opinions. Other cases are normally settled out of court, leaving attorneys and legal scholars without the benefit of publicly available jurisprudence. To give an example of the kind of egregious case that now informs the nascent medical malpractice literature involving use of CAM therapies, in *Johnson v. Tennessee Board of Medical Examiners*,[100] a Tennessee court of appeals upheld a claim for medical malpractice where the defendant physician recommended ozone treatment, administered hydrogen peroxide intravenously, injected vitamin C near the patient's rectum, and treated an abscess with a charcoal poultice mixed in a coffee can.

By way of comparison, in a case involving a non-MD—a chiropractor—the patient came for planar fasciitis in his right heel; the chiropractor fastened a hot pack to the heel, closed the door, and left the room for 12 to 15 minutes.[101] On the chiropractor's return, the patient said, "You're burning the hell out of my foot," whereupon the chiropractor proceeded to apply burn cream to the patient's foot. But it was too late, as the patient needed a skin graft. The patient sued for chiropractic malpractice, and the court upheld the claim, stating that a "reasonably prudent chiropractor" would not have left the room for 12 to 15 minutes with the hot pack on the patient's foot.

Fraud

The tort of fraud is triggered when a health care provider deceives the patient and does so with the intent to so deceive. The deception would have to be intentional and not simply negligent or the result of an honest mistake.

To try to avoid liability for fraud, some healers describe potential results in spiritual rather than physical terms, alluding, again, to the distinction between healing and curing. The argument is that the description of healing work as spiritual helps deflect the perception that the conduct falls within diagnosis and treatment of disease. Courts, however, tend to view medicine broadly as encompassing many forms of healing. They recognize deception with intent to deceive as fraudulent, and are likely to ignore a distinction between healing and curing.

The preceding legal rules provide a preliminary conceptual map for major arenas of misconduct. Taken together, legal rules governing licensing, scope of practice, professional discipline, malpractice, and fraud, do constrain practitioners.

LEGAL ISSUES GOVERNING INSTITUTIONS

Hospitals and other health care institutions should be aware of all five key issues affecting providers of CAM therapies—licensure, scope of practice, professional discipline, malpractice, and fraud. Of these, the first two arenas are relevant to credentialing and quality assurance, while the last three are relevant to potential institutional liability for the negligence of its providers.

Credentialing and Quality Assurance

The Joint Commission on Accreditation of Healthcare Organizations (JCAHO) has a number of rules governing matters such as credentialing and privileging by which JCAHO-accredited hospitals must abide. These rules should be considered when credentialing providers and granting them clinical privileges to deliver CAM therapies. In addition, institutions should avail themselves of the querying process available through the National Practitioner Data Bank.

Institutions and providers often confuse credentialing and privileging. According to JCAHO, credentialing, also known as *credentials review*, means: "the process of obtaining, verifying and assessing the qualifications of a health care practitioner to provide patient care services in or for a health care organization."[102] Privileging, or giving a provider clinical privileges, means: "the process whereby the specific scope and content of patient care services (that is, clinical privileges) are authorized for a health care practitioner by a health care organization based on evaluation of the individual's credentials and performance."[103]

According to JCAHO's *Comprehensive Accreditation Manual for Hospitals*: "All individuals who are permitted by law and by the hospital to provide patient care services independently in the hospital must have delineated clinical privileges, whether or not they are medical staff members."[104] In other words, providers who deliver patient care services independent of medical supervision, and are permitted by their licensing statutes (as well as by hospital rules) to do so, must receive formal clinical privileges. Such privileges typically spell out what procedures the provider may perform. Hospitals have a rigorous internal process to verify the credentials of such providers and ensure that they are qualified and competent to offer such procedures.

Providers who practice dependently (i.e., under the supervision of MDs or DOs), typically go through a similar, but often less rigorous credentialing process, generally outside of the medical staff office and through either their own departments (e.g., physical therapy, nutrition, exercise physiology) or the hospital's Human Resources department. This credentialing process occurs according to established policies and procedures that help the relevant department (or Human Resources) evaluate such matters as training and current competence, media requirements for licensure, and compliance with applicable laws.[105]

Formal clinical privileges, once granted, usually cannot be taken away arbitrarily, as their deprivation is subject to due process rules; and providers who are members of the medical staff also have contractual rights (such as the ability to admit patients to the hospital) and obligations that are delineated in the medical staff bylaws.

In addition to structuring credentialing and privileging decisions, the institution may have other rules applicable to the introduction of CAM therapies. For example, there may be a rule requiring hospital providers to submit any new (CAM) therapies they propose to use through relevant hospital committees (such as a medication use committee if dietary supplements are involved and, potentially, the hospital's Institutional Review Board).

Yet another arena of concern is scope of practice. Institutions should investigate whether providers' own regulatory boards impose any conditions or limitations on use of CAM therapies. For instance, nursing boards in a number of states have addressed the use of CAM therapies as part of legislatively authorized scope of nursing practice.

Institutions, like individual physicians, also should pay attention to the model guidelines promulgated by the Federation of State Medical Boards, mentioned earlier, that aim to govern the practice of CAM therapies by physicians and, particularly, to address issues of deciding what therapies to offer and how to document use of these treatments. As suggested, these guidelines, while they express model rules and have not necessarily been adopted by each state, may exercise influence on the medical board, especially if other regulation in the relevant state is lacking.

Credentialing CAM practitioners generally is similar to credentialing physicians and allied health providers. The essential steps include verification of the following:[106]

- Valid, current state licensure
- Evidence of satisfactory completion of an appropriate national certification examination
- Documentation of completion of required studies and continuing education
- Signed statements pertaining to a specified minimum amount of malpractice insurance
- Documentation of history of malpractice litigation
- Documentation of disciplinary action

The latter two items are included to help the institution determine the extent to which the provider may be a liability risk. Institutions may wish to set standards to help decide whether a certain level or kind of claim in the candidate's history (in either the malpractice or disciplinary arena) is sufficient to disqualify the candidate from consideration. For example, allegations of negligence that have been dismissed by a judge well before trial might be viewed differently than claims involving allegations of sexual abuse that have been aired at a hearing before a professional regulatory board.

Beyond these minimum requirements, institutions seeking a higher level of quality assurance can add criteria such as a preestablished minimum number of years in practice; assessment of practice demographics; letters of recommendation from MDs, DOs and other conventional practitioners to help evaluate how (or how well) the provider has comanaged patients; and assessment through site visits.[107]

Checking the CAM practitioner's credentials, as just outlined, can give the institution some comfort in authorizing the provider to deliver clinical services to patients. As a brief example of how this process might work in the first requirement (valid licensure), consider the case of hiring a massage therapist. Licensing requirements for massage therapists are established by state law in many states and increasingly tend to include a requirement that massage therapists (1) have a minimum of 500 hours of in-class, supervised training at an accredited institution; (2) have passed the national certification examination required by the National Certification Board for Therapeutic Massage and Bodywork; (3) maintain specified continuing education requirements; and (4) carry minimum malpractice insurance.[108]

Many states, however, do not license massage therapists, or simply provide title licensure.[109] In title licensure, the state grants the provider a license to use a specified title (for example, massage therapist) if the provider meets specified educational and training criteria; but unlike mandatory licensure, with title licensure, a provider also may practice without meeting the educational and training prerequisite, provided he or she does not use the specified title.[110] The credentialing process is the same, as the institution still would probably want to hire a massage therapist who is legally authorized to use the title *massage therapist*, but it would be important to pay attention to this legal nuance.

The process of getting the institution to agree in the first place to credential CAM practitioners, and to generate consensus mechanisms to credential such providers, raises different questions. These questions vary by institution, as local politics and preferences regarding CAM therapies vary. We return to this topic in chapter 5.

Potential Institutional Liability

Health care institutions may be liable in malpractice on two theories: direct liability and vicarious liability. Direct liability, which is also known as *corporate negligence*, means that the institution has been directly negligent to the patient. In other words, the health care institution either has done something careless to injure the patient or has carelessly neglected to do something that it should have done, and as a result, the patient has been injured.

Vicarious liability means that the institution has not necessarily done or failed to do something, but rather, becomes liable for the acts of its agents. The law imputes the agent's negligence to the health care institution, the theory being that the hospital is responsible for the agent's conduct.[111] Typically, for example, hospital employees are considered agents of the hospital, and their negligence can be imputed to the hospital. In this way, a single negligent action can give rise to potential liability on both theories of liability: If, for example, a nurse failed to check a patient's vital signs with sufficient regularity in the intensive care unit and the patient died as a result, plaintiff might argue that the hospital was directly negligent for failing to supervise the nurse and also vicariously negligent for the negligence of its employee.

These two theories of liability can apply regardless of whether the institution is offering conventional or CAM therapies, and regardless of whether the provider involved is a conventional or a CAM practitioner. The same principles should, theoretically, apply across the board.

Institutions are the ultimate "deep pockets" for injured patients and thus would benefit from careful consideration of strategy in integrating CAM therapies. Many of the liability and liability management concepts articulated earlier in this chapter also are likely to translate to the institution. For example, since data to date show that there are fewer legal claims against CAM practitioners overall than against medical doctors, there may be fewer such claims against an institution employing CAM practitioners. The risk assessment framework presented later in the book offers health care institutions one possible model for drafting policies about the kinds of therapies they wish to allow (or disallow) and for guiding their conventional health care providers regarding clinical decision making and liability assessment involving CAM therapies.

INSTITUTIONAL FORCES

Besides the legal issues confronting integrative health care centers (IHCs), we seek to understand how and why these centers have developed, what problems they have encountered, how they are responding, and what constitutes success, lack of success, and failure. To analyze and assess the empirical information, we draw on insights offered by several subfields of sociology: the sociology of organizations and institutions, science and knowledge, and medicine and the professions. All of these subfields converge in the study of innovation, a core feature of IHCs. There are no road maps and only a few examples of efforts to develop integrative health care. Among the latter are hospices and palliative care units, both of which have a longer tradition in Britain, for instance, than in the United States. A small literature is emerging in the United States on the development of integrative health care, which includes CAM therapies, in these facilities. For the most part, however, even hospices and palliative care units are innovating as they evolve, placing their efforts within the same frame of reference as the IHCs in our study.

Innovation can be thought of as a process of managing knowledge,[112] a task that becomes necessary when different kinds of knowledge (formal and informal, scientific and everyday, one profession's and another's, one person's and another's, and so on) come into contact. Among the components of knowledge management are gathering and organizing information. Sometimes research produces new information that questions the old. Sometimes patients contribute information that conflicts with a doctor's assumptions. How these various interactions are approached by the key actors in an organization, how differences are meshed and similarities combined, and how parts are aligned to construct wholes, determines whether, for instance, an accommodation occurs that does not radically change the situation or a new product is created that paves the way for broader social change. The act of management itself entails knowledge; it also reflects configurations and struggles involving power and authority.

Clearly, the process of innovation is complex and occurs within multiple, overlapping contexts. IHCs engage in innovation within certain prior parameters, such as environmental constraints and opportunities. Foremost among the contexts shaping the fate of the centers we investigated is the university hospital. From this institutional setting IHCs derive the broad imperative to deliver quality health care within economic strictures. University hospitals also govern the medical and political culture of innovation in IHCs.

At the same time, IHCs develop their own norms of action, influenced in part by the interests and capacities of the main actors involved in the enterprise. The key internal characteristics of IHCs as organizations—size, age, organizational characteristics, leadership styles—are important to establish as baselines of structural differences insofar as they alone may account for differences in efficiency and effectiveness. Other important variables that are more difficult to ascertain include patterns in the exercise of organizational power and capacity to change, and the sources, mechanisms, types and consequences of organizational legitimacy.[113] Understanding the relations of power and authority that regulate IHCs will help to clarify how they legitimize their clinical services and gain the institutional support needed to develop their programs. For example, some centers may be passive actors in the process of institutional development, having received gifts from donors who specify center activities. Others may be more active in developing various sources of support from actors both inside and outside the immediate medical setting. We can hypothesize that these sorts of differences would affect the nature of integrative health care in ways that are to be investigated.

We also assume that the development of an integrative health care center represents an innovation in the hospital or medical center, whether this innovation was generated by dynamic individuals closely affiliated with the center or was the result of a broader process of social change. To further investigate these distinctions, we turn to research on the role of diffusion across organizations to understand how innovative practices spread and structure organizational cultures.[114] By mapping networks of actors and the flow of ideas, we can investigate the extent to which developments in integrative health care rest on a self-contained system of ideas and support or involve contact with actors, ideas, and organizations outside the immediate medical community. We would hypothesize that IHCs would gain strength from developing a wider network of affiliations that enable them to engage in more continual processes of legitimating their endeavor. Thus, we can understand similarities and differences among the IHCs to be based less on conventional organizational features than on networks of organizational culture.

From the perspective of the sociology of science we can appreciate that medicine is a social institution that has a distinctive set of norms and values and, much like other social institutions, both affects and is affected by its social and cultural contexts.[115] At present the scientific medical community requires that innovations in health care be proved through scientific research before they are implemented in practice. To this end, the National Center for Complementary and Alternative Medicine (NCCAM) and the National Institutes of Health (NIH) funded a number of studies on the safety and efficacy of various CAM modalities. We evaluate the significance of this research in informing the clinical activities of the center, hypothesizing that if the centers are cognizant of research findings and largely guided by them, their capacity to legitimize their endeavors may be enhanced.

However, we also expected and did find that some IHCs are not significantly influenced by the research on CAM, or that the weight of evidenced-based practice is less substantial than some other factors. When this occurred, we sought to discover what other factors overshadowed the findings of current research on CAM, and hypothesized that these centers would have a more local culture, in which knowledge is "manufactured" in accordance with social and political peculiarities.[116] For example, a primary reliance on one particular CAM therapy may occur when a powerful individual in a leadership position pursues a personal agenda.

Furthermore, we expected to and did find variations in the practice and understanding of "integrative" across the centers. These too, we felt, could be explained in terms of the local culture of the IHC. For instance, suppose one center insists that the application of a particular CAM therapy occur after conventional treatment, while another center employs the same therapy at the same time or even before conventional treatment. Such variations would support the hypotheses of some sociologists of science who claim that scientific inquiry (understood here as knowledge about CAM) is situationally contingent and determined by the ideologies and interests, rewards and punishments, statuses and power relations among layers of social, political, and economic factors in the lives of clinicians. It is important to discern whether science or other factors are driving developments in CAM and to specify what these other factors might be. This analysis can inform other integrative centers regarding the variables that will drive the clinical model of integration they wish to pursue.

The medical profession in the United States has weathered the intrusion of several government regulatory measures, prepaid group health plans in the private sector, increasing malpractice insurance rates, scrutiny from all sides, demands for improved accountability, and much more.[117] It has survived, but it has also experienced unprecedented change in its social status and political legitimacy.[118] Its ability to control the terms of occupational practices—the defining characteristic of any profession—has diminished, along with its autonomy in medical decision making. The introduction of CAM therapies into American health care is seen by some segments of the medical profession as one more in a long series of efforts to undermine professional integrity, indeed as a harbinger of "demedicalization" let alone "deprofessionalization." But a larger and ever-growing number of physicians understand that CAM promises an opportunity for innovation in health care as well as a venue for renewing the profession's ability to communicate with patients. In short, CAM has the potential to humanize medicine.[119] What binds these groups together is the insistence that CAM be evidence based. It remains to be seen whether the development of IHCs can help to blur, if not dissolve, the division within the medical profession on the role of CAM in the future of health care.

Despite the movement toward a more favorable medical and political landscape, social obstacles to integrative care persist, slowing and, in some cases, halting the evolution from the dominance of conventional medicine toward a model that integrates conventional medicine and CAM therapies. Integrative care also raises issues of dominance and hegemony, including questions as to whether medical doctors will need to supervise various CAM practitioners, and which providers (conventional or CAM) will be the gatekeepers through whom patients are referred to others within the same group practice or setting. The pioneering struggles and successes, fights and failures, obstacles and opportunities, presented in our study may offer models for other clinics and institutions that are moving individualized experiments in integrative care through their own institutional processes.

CHAPTER 4

Starting Up and Growing

Overcoming Hurdles and
Developing Sustainability

ORIGINS AND GROWTH

Innovation in hospital and health care services is a slow and protracted process. The introduction of integrative health may be seen as an exception. When we consider that the American Medical Association did not dissolve its Committee on Quackery until 1990 and that rigorous, scientific investigations of CAM therapies were not fully underway until the late 1990s, it is remarkable that as many as 15% of the hospitals surveyed by the American Hospital Association in 2001, cited earlier, were offering at least one CAM therapy. Although there are no data on growth across the United States, we know that increasingly more CAM provision is becoming institutionalized within integrative healthcare centers (IHCs). Certainly increased institutionalization is suggested by such trends as the growing number of studies testifying to widespread consumer use of CAM therapies; the increasing attention to policy and practice (as evidenced by the reports by the White House Commission and Institute of Medicine, among others); and the growth of interinstitutional bodies (such as the Consortium of Academic Health Centers for Integrative Medicine,[120] an increasingly numerous body of academic medical centers[121] whose mission is "to help transform medicine and healthcare through rigorous scientific studies, new models of clinical care, and innovative educational programs that integrate biomedicine, the complexity of human beings, the intrinsic nature of healing and the rich diversity of therapeutic systems."

This chapter presents the overall characteristics of the 23 IHCs we studied in depth. Appendix C summarizes their main features. Many of these IHCs have undergone major structural changes (one center is in its third iteration); some because of earlier problems, some because of seemingly capricious changes in or by hospital leadership. However, the success of other IHCs is driving major expansion. Although the centers are at various stages of development, vary in size, level, and kind of funding, and much else, they are experiencing a common set of challenges. As we discuss their experiences, we present at the same time the reasons for the challenges and the diversity in center responses. We also elucidate the meaning and practice of integration. Insofar as all of the IHCs in our study are affiliated with hospitals, we will see that the role of conventional medicine is critical to the operation of each center. In many ways, how each center implements its vision of integration depends on the climate of support at each institution. Nevertheless, the commonalities that are emerging in the practice of integration are as important as the differences. The delicate balance between giving patients what they want and guiding them to make informed choices—that is, autonomy versus paternalism—as well as the balance between market factors and medical decision making is evident in the institutionalization of IHCs. How to convince hospital administrators and physicians of the value of these centers, how to decide which therapists to employ, and how to maintain financial solvency are among the many questions IHCs presently face.

THE CENTERS

We focused on IHCs affiliated with academic medical centers because these would strive, we felt, for the highest quality of care and represent state-of-the-art mainstream thinking about such issues as regulation. The IHCs in our study are at various stages of development, all are subject to regular Joint Commission on Accreditation of Healthcare Organizations (JCAHO) reviews, their sizes range from 3 to 25 full time equivalent (FTEs), and they service anywhere up to 1,500 patients per month (some of whom visit more than once a week). Some of the clinics have their own facilities in the hospital or some other location in the medical center, others share physical space with another unit, in one case a community clinic. One university decided to construct a virtual center with several satellite locations and activities as a way of avoiding cost and institutional commitment. Some of the centers are affiliated with a department at the medical school; some have undergone changes in affiliation due to lack of support by the initial parent department or unit. One director noted that being in a department both sheltered and limited the center. She and others expressed hope that their center would become a self-contained division, enabling them to spread their affiliations across a number of departments. In this way, the center not only shifts the scene or ground over turf battles but also disseminates the idea of integrative medicine more widely. Many centers already have ongoing working relations across several units, even if their parent location is circumscribed.

The Idea

As we have noted, surveys of CAM use among Americans indicate significant growth in the last 15 years. Consumer interest is by far the major driving force behind the expansion of CAM services in a variety of venues across the US, including hospitals. Nearly half of the hospitals surveyed by the American Hospital Association in 2001 reported that patient demand was the primary motivation for offering CAM services.[122] In a few of the centers in our study, either the dean of the medical school or a member of the hospital board became aware of growing interest in CAM among patients or within the community. Recognizing an opportunity to make the hospital more visible and the desire and need to attract more patients, these individuals discussed the idea of offering CAM services with other administrators or board members and, above all, with physicians at the hospital.

Surveys have also shown increasingly more receptive attitudes among physicians toward CAM. Once again, the reason for this development rests squarely on the use of CAM by patients, who in many cases want to discuss their use with physicians and perhaps ask for advice. The gap between physicians' knowledge and the needs and desires of patients has led a growing number of physicians to attend continuing medical education courses on CAM and to purchase textbooks on CAM designed for practicing and physicians-in-training. Major medical schools across the country are offering these courses, using the new textbooks available in CAM and integrative medicine, and are finding increasing demand for them. However, surveys have also shown that many patients are not telling their physicians about their use of CAM, indicating not only a barrier in communications but also a strain in physician–patient relations. Awareness of this disjuncture has prompted physicians to want to learn more about CAM and how to better discuss these and related issues with patients.

A few of the IHCs in our study were the brainchild of physicians, or in some cases, researchers or nurses. Through casual conversations, these individuals sought each other out. They gathered informally or in meetings to discuss their common interests and strategize on the next steps they could take to further their ideas. They determined, through surveys, e-mails, or notices, the extent of need, interest, and demand at the hospital.

In many cases, they discovered more interest and demand than they expected. This networking brought a number of individuals, who had been engaged with CAM in some way for years, out of their autonomous existence. Eventually, groups of interested individuals approached department chairs, deans, and hospital administrators for advice and guidance. If hospital board members were not already part of these efforts, their approval was sought. One of the centers in our study was empowered to set up a task force of 50 that included community representatives; together they constructed a strategic plan. In those centers where the idea initiated at the level of researchers and nurses, the process of garnering wider support usually took at least a year, sometimes 2 or 3 years. Once physicians were included among the participants, the process of evolution to the next stages was quicker and smoother. Since deans are generally physicians themselves, once they were convinced, it was relatively easy for them to bring other physicians on board.

Funding

Although these scenarios occurred in some form in all of the centers in our study, many began because of the special interest of a private donor. Rarely did these individuals have a clear idea of what they wanted. For most, a positive experience with CAM, either personally or through a close relative or friend, inspired a philanthropic spirit. In a few cases, donors placed restrictions on the use of funds (making them time-limited, specifying that they could be used only for certain purposes). In addition, some donors suggested a greater emphasis on either research efforts or clinical activities. Some also required matching funds from the university or hospital. In no case was the initial funding (whether from one donor or a number of donations) sufficiently large to establish a full-service IHC without the need for additional fund-raising. In many cases, the donations were small and covered only start-up activities.

In a typical scenario, a physician in one hospital spent years gathering support for her vision and, at the same time, raising funds for its inception. This center, which she now directs, was the result of "thousands of small donations." Its expansion has required more of the same. Less typical is the experience of another director, whose center is in a major urban area where residents generously support a wide range of activities. She found fund-raising to be relatively easy, and managed to raise sufficient funds so that the affiliated hospital did not have to contribute more than infrastructure support. She was also able to take the time to develop a full-fledged IHC.

A handful of IHCs are funded primarily, if not solely, by the hospital or academic center, relieving them of the burden of fund-raising. The extent of financial commitment varies considerably. In one case, the administration has been remarkably generous due, in large part, to patient demand; it pays the full cost of certain therapies provided to inpatients and their families. In most of the other IHCs, activities are limited and administrations, while supportive, are taking a wait-and-see approach to the possibility of expansion of support. Some hospitals or universities cover the operating costs of IHCs; others provide infrastructure support but no actual funding.

The Mission

Once they agreed to pursue the idea, hospital boards and administrators generally decided to recruit an MD to translate vision into reality, direct the development of business plans, and eventually direct the IHC. In a few cases, individuals with PhDs became center directors, but MDs were always on hand to oversee clinical activities and function as medical directors.[123] The inclusion of MDs is an important feature of the IHCs in our study. Although patient demand may have introduced CAM to health care providers, the legitimacy of integrative medicine rests first and foremost on its subsequent acceptance by the medical profession. Indeed, evolution of the terms used to label CAM—from alternative to complementary to integrative—implies a process of winning the hearts and minds of physicians. In all of the IHCs we studied, CAM is an adjunct to conventional medicine. The presence of physicians, as clinical or medical directors if not always center directors, means that medical conditions receive attention first, before CAM therapies are used, and they are monitored as CAM treatment proceeds. The mission of these centers is to offer patients the best of both CAM and conventional medicine. If they did not actually say these or similar words in mission statements printed on their brochures, most of the center directors and staff agreed with the following definition on the meaning of integration:

> Integrative medicine is not simply concerned with giving physicians new tools, such as herbs in addition to or instead of pharmaceutical drugs. Rather it aims to shift some of the basic orientations of medicine: toward healing rather than symptomatic treatment, toward a closer relationship with nature, toward a strengthened doctor–patient relationship and an emphasis on mind and spirit in addition to body.

However, in practice, as we will see, the types of integration that occur depend on a number of factors related to both the patient and the center itself.

All of the centers wanted to present themselves as closely tied to conventional medicine and to dispel in advance any impressions that some physicians harbor linking CAM or wellness with boutique health care. Some centers had to overcome an earlier incarnation as a spa or dissociate themselves from spas connected with the hospital.

The Business Plan

Insofar as the IHCs in our study are affiliated with academic centers as well as hospitals, they can encompass three different types of programs: clinical services, research activities, and education. Although the business plan pertains primarily to the clinic, all three functions could involve a financial component. Most of the center directors decided to start small, limiting either the inclusion of all three programs, their scope, the variety of therapies or conditions included, or all of these. All of the centers in our study had clinical programs, but some had no or minimal research and/or education programs.

With regard to clinical services, many directors decided to contain their ambitions and, as one director said, "grow organically, according to demand and ability to cover costs." For the most part, these centers focused on outpatient services only. At the most minimal level, some centers maintain a list of CAM practitioners in the community to whom they can "refer" patients. In fact, a few directors indicated that their goal was to support, and not to compete, with what already exists in the community, implying that they may not develop a service-based clinic. In some cases, clinics draw from community practitioners who spend some days at the university clinic and other days of the week in their private community practices. At another level, some centers screen patients and offer advice but few if any therapies per se. At a higher level, some centers have facilities where they offer a limited number of therapies. Maximally, a few centers offer a wide range of therapies in specialized clinics. Some centers have also developed inpatient services; others are planning this extension of their programs within a few years. Only a few centers that focus on specific illnesses offer therapies primarily to inpatients.

Research plays a special role within many of the centers but its importance varies considerably among them. The directors or others at many centers either engage in research themselves or reach out to medical school faculty who might be interested in conducting research on CAM through the center. Directors continually seek to identify faculty who are interested in researching CAM, recruit them to participate in the center's activities, and convince them to use the center in some way in their research, most frequently by running their grants through the center. In some cases, IHCs forged a new integration among the faculty interested in or already conducting research on CAM. Elsewhere, center directors, codirectors, or others on the staff were already conducting research on

CAM and transferred at least part of their grants to the center. Clearly, research is a critical source of funds for many of the centers. And it carries the intangible bonus of legitimacy. However, a number of the center directors complained about university or hospital policies on the division of overhead from grants. Since all research faculty have departmental appointments, many departments or another branch of the medical school expect to receive a significant portion of the overhead.

The importance placed on educational offerings also varies. A number of centers lack the scope and depth to accommodate physician training; a few centers stress their centrality to fostering the national direction of integrative medicine. Some centers receive grants to train MDs (commonly from one of the primary care specialties) as fellows, who learn formally and informally, through research or continuing education courses, on either a part-time or full-time basis, about integrative medicine at the centers. Most IHCs allow or encourage residents to include the clinic in their rotations. MDs at the IHC may also teach CAM courses at the medical school. Inclusion in the required medical curriculum is difficult. All of the centers engaged in some sort of public education and outreach activities, at the least offering brochures and other information on CAM therapies, at the most, providing a library, computers, or regularly scheduled classes with both lectures and activities.

A few IHCs in our study have sought to integrate all of the CAM services being provided at their hospital and all of the CAM research being conducted at their university. In some cases, this integration has brought all CAM-related activities under one roof, but in most it has resulted in a network of contacts. One committee that investigated the range of CAM activities at its university decided to maintain a virtual integrative medicine center, enabling satellites to develop specific activities in depth, while remaining cognizant of activities elsewhere through periodic meetings of the whole. However, a number of the IHCs in our study have not pursued integration among the faculty or have not been able to achieve it. The reasons are often political, reflecting issues of turf—at the level of departments or centers and related to grants or prestige. Some of these latter directors resent the unsystematic approach to CAM and, recognizing their own impotence, can only hope that their universities create a superstructure to more truly integrate CAM and conventional medicine.

CHOOSING THERAPIES AND PRACTITIONERS

One of the most important decisions that directors have to make is which therapies to offer and which practitioners to hire. For a number of directors, the decision was based on their own research interests or those of affiliated faculty at the hospital. In the same vein, many of the centers in our study conducted surveys in their affiliated hospitals to find out if any physicians or nurses were themselves CAM practitioners and which therapies hospital personnel and patients were most interested in. Several directors were surprised at the extent of untapped resources and unfulfilled demand: physicians who were acupuncturists or practiced biofeedback, nurses who were energy healers or massage therapists, hospital staff who wanted relaxation or yoga classes.

Whether or not a core of CAM capacity and interest was already present, directors weighed a number of factors in deciding which therapies to offer. One medical director struck a common chord in articulating three criteria in her decision: (1) what the community wants, balanced against (2) what the medical profession thinks is credible (that is, evidence-based therapies), and (3) practitioner availability (see chapter 1). Another director added a fourth factor closely related to the second—politics. With regard to the first, only a few of the centers had the resources to survey the larger community to assess interest; others engaged in informal techniques to gather information about local interests. However, all of the directors in our study consulted published surveys on the use of CAM to gain some sense of the more widely used therapies not only across the country but also among regional and local populations.

Determining the evidence base was much more direct. There is a growing literature on the safety and efficacy of a wide variety of CAM therapies. Funded in significant part by the NCCAM, research using randomized controlled clinical trials is not only sorting the wheat from the chaff in CAM therapies, but also providing clinicians with specific information about the types of disorders most likely to benefit from a particular type of treatment. Mainstream medical journals as well as peer-reviewed CAM journals regularly publish research findings. There is now a sufficient number of published research studies that one journal specializes in publishing only reviews of large numbers of research studies on given topics in CAM and integrative medicine. However, the extent to which the research is directing choice of CAM therapy must be taken with a grain of salt. One director admitted that experiential, rather than experimental, evidence sufficed. She said that her hospital was patient oriented. So, if patients feel that massage improves their quality of life, they will receive massage—barring adverse consequences.

All of the centers sought practitioners who were credentialed and licensed according to the requirements in their state. Beyond legal frameworks, some hospitals require that patients with certain illnesses (such as cancer) obtain physicians' orders before they receive certain CAM therapies (acupuncture, yoga, full-body massage, physical therapy). Also, some states require referrals for certain practitioners. Problems regarding credentialing and licensing arise for the most part with those therapies, such as mind–body relaxation techniques and movement therapies, which have variable standards. Where there were no guidelines in place, center directors consulted local, state, or national organizations to gather information about standards for qualifications and registration. In some centers, relaxation therapies are conducted by nurses or, in a few cases, MDs, whose credentials allow them to include additional practices without specific licensing. Some massage therapists also use such practices as Reiki, which may or may not fall within their legislatively authorized scope of practice.[124] A number of the IHCs in our study have practitioners or health workers who do more than one therapy. Often these include the more loosely regulated mind–body therapies. A special problem arose in centers that employed acupuncturists who were MDs in China but are not recognized as MDs in the United States, raising questions about their scope of practice. Because most states have rules regarding acupuncturists, these cases can generally be readily resolved. Issues of credentialing, licensing, and scope of practice are elaborated in chapter 5.

In addition to practice qualifications, all directors sought prospective therapists who were committed to teamwork and the idea of integrated health care. Some centers also sought affinity with their philosophy—for example, an emphasis on the role of the spirit in healing. One director emphasized that, because practitioners would be dealing with physicians, they needed to be conversant and comfortable with the medical model as well as willing and able to refrain from using their own CAM terminology. Another director said she did not have to advertise—"once word got out [prospective practitioners] were beating down our doors."

There is an interesting consistency across our centers in therapies offered. The most frequently available are acupuncture and massage, the two big ticket items, as well as mind–body (relaxation) therapies. There are also a number of practitioners who are barely considered to be CAM practitioners insofar as their fields were mainstreamed years ago: osteopath, psychologist, physical therapist, nutritionist, or dietician. However, what these practitioners do in the setting of an IHC may be different than what they do in private practice or in other practice settings.

The politics of acceptability refers most strongly to two therapies—chiropractic and homeopathy—which we expected would be relatively absent from the centers. We were wrong. Regarding the former, even though the literature shows that chiropractic is the most frequently used practitioner-based CAM therapy, it is also the most politically unacceptable. Availability of chiropractic care is correlated to the relatively large number and wide distribution of chiropractors relative to other CAM practitioners (chapter 1) There is also an increasing body of evidence regarding the safety, effectiveness and cost-effectiveness of chiropractic care for low back pain, the most common cause of disability in working Americans.[21]

The legacy of litigation by the American Medical Association, and counterlitigation by the chiropractic profession (such as the antitrust case, *Wilks vs. AMA*), has left its mark on the medical establishment, which "has not yet fully accepted chiropractic as a mainstream form of medical care."[125] However, almost all states now have legislation requiring that insurers include chiropractors. Their changing status is also reflected in their relatively high number in the IHCs we studied.

Homeopathy is more widely used in Europe, where it is licensed and reimbursed under national health care systems, than in the United States. American physicians are somewhat disdainful of the inability to scientifically prove the mechanisms of action of homeopathy, insofar as its dilution too closely approximates water.[126] In our study, centers with naturopaths were more likely to offer homeopathy.

One other therapy, herbal remedies, raises thorny issues for center directors. Because the Food and Drug Administration does not require botanicals to show evidence of efficacy prior to marketing and distribution, physicians may be reluctant to recommend them. Our interviews revealed that many center directors are reluctant even to discuss herbs because of the perceived paucity of scientific proof of safety and efficacy. Some of the larger IHCs in our study have hired nutritionists who include consideration of herbal supplements when counseling patients. In many states, the use of herbs by acupuncturists who are also traditional Chinese medicine practitioners falls in a gray area. In general, centers with an interest in herbs allow their practitioners to recommend them. Two centers in our study plan to stock and sell herbs in the near future. Some center directors admitted to being encumbered by the Pharmaceutical and Therapeutics Committees of their affiliated hospitals; most committees only allow center staff to discuss herbs.

A more complete (but not exhaustive) list of the therapies offered across the centers includes: acupuncture, traditional Chinese medicine (or Oriental medicine), nutritional counseling, herbal counseling, naturopathy, homeopathy, osteopathy, chiropractic, physical therapy, yoga, Tai Chi, Qi Gong, massage, Shiatsu, therapeutic touch, Reiki, biofeedback, hypnosis, psychotherapy, mindfulness meditation, guided imagery, mind–body (not specified), expressive arts therapy, music therapy, and pastoral care.

DELIVERING CARE

When Patients First Come to the Center

Most patients who visit the IHCs in our study are self-referred, having heard about the center through word of mouth or the center's community outreach efforts. Although health care workers may also be among patients' sources of information, most of them do not actually refer; they may recommend or suggest, however. Nevertheless, a number of physicians are beginning to refer their patients to IHCs, generally when reimbursement or managed care issues are involved or because their patients have special medical disorders or health care needs. Overall, centers in our study receive about one-third of their patients through physician referrals. Only a few require referrals for all patients. Some centers require that patients with particular medical conditions receive formal approval from their physicians before receiving certain CAM treatments—acupuncture, full-body, deep (but not necessarily light) massage, movement therapies, and herbs. Generally the mind–body therapies are not subject to physician approval. Many of the center directors in our study expressed the hope and expectation that physician referrals would increase as word about the IHC spread in their local areas and as knowledge about CAM increased.

The role of the clinical director is to ensure that patients with medical disorders receive appropriate treatment and to communicate with primary care or specialist physicians about this treatment. In the case of inpatients, the formality and intensity of consultations with specialists vary depending on the therapy and the condition of the patient. Some hospitals allow verbal consent by the specialist. In all cases, someone (the therapist, a nurse, or the physician) records the treatment on the patient's chart. Outpatients who do not have medical disorders are usually encouraged to see a primary care physician (PCP) outside the center. Some centers require that all patients have a PCP; others require that patients see a PCP by their third visit to the IHC. In a few centers in our study, having a PCP is necessary only for those patients with medical disorders, and medical exams are required only for those patients who have not had one within the last several years. A few of the centers represented here offer primary care when necessary or requested, but most prefer that patients receive primary care outside of the IHC. Communication between the IHC and the PCP varies. Physicians and, in the case of patients with no medical problem, non-MD practitioners at the centers commonly take the initiative to contact primary care or specialist physicians regarding a patient's care. One director told us that she tries to send reports to every health care provider involved in a patient's care.

Centers explicitly develop these policies to assuage any concerns within hospitals and academic centers about patients receiving "proper" care. At the least, all CAM practitioners have a duty to refer to an MD any patient who has a medical complaint that raises issues beyond the practitioner's expertise and training.[127]

In a few centers patients see either the medical director or another physician or a team of MDs and practitioners at the outset to develop individualized programs. Many of the IHCs use a nurse for the initial patient screening and sometimes triage. Patients can also book appointments for consultations with an MD or nurse at the center. A few of the centers limit their practice to consultations in which MDs (individually or as a team) assess patients, acquaint them with the variety of therapies relevant to their needs or desires, and guide them to make appropriate choices. These centers generally keep a list of community practitioners, whether or not they actually refer or recommend that patients see any particular practitioners. In general, however, when patients come to an IHC, they tend to see whichever CAM practitioner they want without triage or consultation. In this case, it is "up to the practitioner to decide if their therapy is the right one for the patient," said one director. But all of the centers record in some way the medical histories of all patients. In some centers all of the practitioners are credentialed to take medical histories. Some, but not all, of the medical directors (who may or not be the center or clinical director) sign off on treatment plans for patients without medical problems. For the most part, centers require patients to sign informed consent releases only before receiving the more invasive therapies (acupuncture, perhaps full-body massage). A few centers require these for all treatments.

To some extent, these differences in the delivery of care occur because of differences in the extent of illness in the client/patient population. A few small centers with limited capacity accept only well patients. In general, patients who are less sick tend to direct their own health care. Some directors felt they were criticized for being too wellness oriented. Insofar as a number of private sector hospitals are aggressively developing wellness or spalike facilities, the academic setting of the IHCs in our study most likely accounts for these dismissive attitudes.

CAM Practitioners

Many of the MDs and nurses at IHCs are themselves CAM practitioners. A few of the smaller IHCs are staffed entirely by health care workers (or social workers) already at the hospital. Although issues of salary, credentialing, and so on are simpler with these individuals, their work at the centers is not problem-free. MDs in particular have to negotiate with their departments on such issues as how much time they can commit to the centers.

Generally, at least one staff person is in full-time attendance at the centers; the time commitment of the others varies. The majority of practitioners are independent contractors who work at the IHC on a part-time basis. One director admitted that there is not enough demand for certain practitioners to be at the center full-time. Most of the practitioners have private practices in addition to their work at the IHC. Many of them would like to increase the number of hours they work at the centers, to make them eligible for benefits and also because they enjoy the ambience and quality of the work setting. Most directors also noted that their preference was to increase the hours of current practitioners before hiring others and diversifying the therapies offered, adding that practitioners who do not receive benefits would thereby become eligible.

By and large, centers pay practitioners on a fee-for-service basis, with rates that are standard in the community. In a number of cases, the center takes a percentage of these fees for overhead, so in general, the fees are inflated to reflect the center's share. In most centers, the fees vary by practitioner. However, one director told us that all of the practitioners in her center charge the same fee for their services. Another director noted that certain therapists could make more money in private practice, implying that practitioners are not in IHCs for the income alone. In a few centers, practitioners are salaried, but patients are charged on a fee-for-service basis. Directors indicated that the salary format enables centers to pay practitioners on a more regular and equitable basis (assuming that practitioners work the same number of hours). They also said that while fees provide an incentive to see more clients, salaries offer the luxury of time for staff meetings, research, and more informal interaction among practitioners. In only rare centers are practitioners fully salaried. Some centers have a mix of salaried and independent contractor practitioners.

Most IHC directors work closely with hospital lawyers on contract, scope of practice, and risk management issues and on developing protocols for such questions as contraindications, record-keeping requirements, and determining when people are and are not patients (generally, if they are being treated for specific medical conditions, such as back pain, they are officially patients). These precautions as well as the insistence that the centers and their practitioners are following evidence-based practices exist not only for legal reasons. They are also central to relations between IHCs and their affiliated hospital physicians, who are concerned about such matters.

In all of the centers the medical director provides the safety net below which patients will not fall, whether or not she actually sees a patient or discusses the patient's care with the practitioner. In a number of centers, practitioners work relatively independently, deciding on their own when questions beyond their competence arise and require them to approach the medical director. Said one medical director, "It is up to the medical director to pick practitioners who know [what patients need] and to know how to do what is needed," including consulting the medical director. At a minimum, medical directors review patients' charts.

Most of the medical directors indicated that they try to keep close watch over practitioners to ensure that they are maintaining regular standards of practice and keeping up with new developments in their fields. However, while there is some supervision everywhere, levels vary. One practitioner told us that she regularly reports to her mentor in the department of medicine, but she doubted that the center director monitored the other practitioners much, despite the yearly evaluations. One medical director said that she does "not go to the [practitioners] to make sure they know about [new studies];" she is "not constantly checking up on what [practitioners] do." This director can maintain her level of trust because she meets regularly with practitioners in team meetings where she can convey her expectations. All medical directors check patients' charts, but these too vary from random and every few months to systematic and weekly. The former tends to occur in centers that have weekly case conferences or that have primarily well patients, the latter in centers specializing in specific illnesses.

Policies regarding the treatment of inpatients also differ among centers that offer this service. In one center, although practitioners are credentialed to provide inpatient services, they do not and probably will not because the center is planning to retain an in-hospital staff of CAM practitioners. In another center, which has become independent from both the hospital and the university, the hospital reimburses the center for inpatient services. Staff members of a third center, which provides only a limited range of inpatient therapies, help these patients find outside practitioners who are paid privately on a fee-for-service basis. Because these services are strictly private, no physician referral is needed.

WORKING RELATIONS—INTERNAL DYNAMICS

How centers deliver services, especially how practitioners at the centers interact with physicians outside it, represents one dimension of the practice of integration. In addition, integration refers to how physicians and CAM practitioners who work in the centers relate to and interact with each other, and how patients are included in these interactions. Our findings indicate that although integration is an evolving experience, grounded in the situational specificities of each center, there are some significant commonalities. However, there are also revealing inconsistencies among the IHCs we studied. Some of these variations pertain to organizational features of the center; others are due to differences among patients—the nature of their illness, their stated needs and desires, their network of health care providers. But most are the result of the culture of integration that has been created by everyone involved with the center.

To unravel the meaning and practice of integration, let us begin with the role of the patient. When a patient self-refers to a particular practitioner and sees no one else, it may well be that the patient is doing her own integrating by deciding which practitioner to see, when to visit her PCP, and what to say to her various health care providers. Insofar as CAM elevates patient participation and responsibility, the extent of integration is ultimately up to patients. Frequently, however, patients work with practitioners in making decisions about treatment. One director emphasized to us her center's "focus on developing ongoing, consultative mechanisms to help patients identify their needs and engage in self-healing." While this center offers some mind–body and movement therapies, it mostly functions, at present, as a central referral system for community practitioners. In several centers in our study, the first practitioner a patient chooses to see becomes responsible for integrating care. Together with the patient, this practitioner decides how long treatment should last, whether additional therapies might be helpful or other therapies better suited to the patient's needs, whether to communicate with physicians, and so on. Theoretically, it is possible to say, as did one director, that any practitioner proficient in more than one therapy or an MD who is also a CAM practitioner "integrates" themselves. But the truer spirit of integration goes beyond these minimalist forms.

In a few of the centers in our study, the clinical or medical director plays a central role in the practice of integration. These directors regularly discuss a patient's care with both the practitioner(s) and the patient to decide on treatment options and coordination. The importance of having both medical and CAM input in the practice of integration prompted one clinical director (an RN) to question this feature in her clinic, where "it's either the medical director or the staff primary MD that does the integrating. The practitioners tend to do their thing and then leave." In contrast, some directors expressed the view that the need for integration arises when patients see more than one CAM practitioner; that is, integration may not include conventional medicine. We found significant variation on what, exactly, medical or clinic directors did, either to be integrators themselves or to oversee the integrative functions of practitioners and patients.

Arguably, the fullest extent of integration occurs in centers that hold weekly or monthly case conferences at which practitioners meet as a group to discuss certain patients (usually those with more difficult or complicated illnesses or personal situations), with their permission. In addition to institutionalized meetings and team conferences, in some centers practitioners make a point of informal interaction, whether to talk about patients or issues. Although these interactions are by nature random, IHCs develop norms that are created by the practitioners themselves as well as by the tone set by the director and the facilitation for interaction she fashions. Although all of the directors lauded interaction among practitioners on a regular basis as ideal, we noted that its occurrence is happenstance if it is not systematized. In some centers, these regular meetings are enriched by occasionally inviting guest lecturers. In some centers, many practitioners are reluctant to participate in group meetings because it takes away from time with clients and is not reimbursed.

A different form of integration occurs in those few IHCs that assign a team leader for each patient or each therapy. A few of the people we interviewed voiced yet one additional feature of integration. One clinical director (an RN) complained that it was a problem having a medical director who was a specialist, because the therapies used tended to reflect her orientation and interests, thereby making the clinic less integrative. In a similar vein, another director (an MD) felt that her center was not very integrative because only a narrow range of therapies was offered. Finally, some centers achieved a virtual type of integration by providing practitioners access to electronic medical records enabling them to, if not coordinate care, at least see what other therapies patients are receiving. In a few centers only MDs had access to these records.

THE BROADER NETWORK: POLITICS AND PATIENCE

Good relations with hospital physicians may be an important contributor to the success of an IHC. One of the first reports published by the Office of Alternative Medicine at the National Institutes of Health (NIH) predicted that "belief barriers," that is, credibility on the part of the medical community precluded greater adoption of CAM within conventional medical settings.[128] Indeed, a survey by the American Hospital Association found that physician resistance was the major obstacle facing hospitals in implementing successful CAM programs.[129] Personnel in all of the centers in our study were fully aware of these challenges and fully attuned to the political pulse of their institutions. All of the directors have been astute in paving their paths toward acceptance.

A priority task for the center director is introducing hospital MDs to the science and efficacy of CAM. Many directors who are themselves MDs conduct grand rounds to explain how a particular therapy or cluster of therapies can be used as an adjunct in the care of patients with particular illnesses or disorders. The emphasis here is on two ideas: CAM is a complement, not an alternative, to medical treatment, and specific types of CAM therapies are used for specific disorders. To support the latter, center directors have to be cognizant of the research on CAM. In describing the stance they adopted toward CAM when talking with hospital physicians, directors told us they assumed open-mindedness on the part of their audience but were careful not to appear to be advocates of CAM themselves.

However, one director acknowledged that the doctors in her hospital were "not impressed with the studies" on CAM, even though these were conducted through randomized, controlled trial (RCT)s and explained mechanisms of action. She added that physicians "are oriented to clinical experience. By and large they are not quantitatively oriented so meta-analyses don't mean much. They know aspirin helps even though there have been no studies [sic]." Another director was more sanguine about the change that had developed among her colleagues, noting that she "does not hear physicians saying [CAM] is bogus," as was the case in the past.

The following summary scenarios both capture the problems of communicating about CAM and handling the concerns of hospital physicians, and also offer suggestions for how other directors might approach the issues. One director (not the only one) in our study took several years to build support with hospital physicians ("to overcome institutional bias," said another director) through direct communication. Since she already had credibility and stature as a surgeon at the hospital, she had a strong foundation to transform personal relations into clinical open-mindedness. (Another director noted that MDs will only listen to MDs on the subject of CAM.) Once the funds for the IHC were in place, she identified both converts and lingering skeptics among the hospital physicians and invited both to be members of the initial steering committee. She continues to invite physicians to weekly case conferences. Hers is perhaps the riskiest route to winning physician acceptance, but it also holds the most promise for success.

Another director engages in considerable networking. As center plans were being developed, she went to every department in the hospital to explain the center—its purpose, how it would work, how physicians could use it. She continues to visit as many departments as possible and also makes a point of sitting on hospital committees. As with the previous director, she too felt that establishing trust through personal relations was imperative.

Another director who came to a setting where there had been considerable skepticism about CAM emphasized the importance of going slowly in building personal relations and introducing physicians to CAM. Besides conducting grand rounds, she also found it useful to develop a small-scale program that makes certain CAM therapies (massage, reflexology, aromatherapy) available to inpatients in a particular unit. Because nurses are the main link with physicians, gaining their support and assistance with this program and working with the physicians to set it up have been invaluable. This director also works with hospital units to develop wellness regimens for patients after discharge.

In addition to developing personal relations, most of the centers in our study were actively seeking to develop collaborations with their affiliated hospitals and universities, whether these were related to education or research or both. Some directors voiced the opinion that physicians would only become more open-minded about CAM through direct involvement with the center.

These and similar efforts are radically transforming the climate of working relations between the medical profession and IHCs. Although there are still pockets of resistance, a number of directors in the centers that have been operating more than 2 years reported remarkable progress in winning physician interest and approval.

THE BOTTOM LINE: FINANCIAL VIABILITY

For the most part, hospital administrators have remained supportive of center efforts, both morally and financially. Some directors indicated gratitude for the "tremendous" support they were receiving. Elsewhere the administration's stance was more lukewarm and tentative. These variations aside, the vast majority of IHC directors have begun to feel an increasing pressure to prove that the centers can be self-sustaining, which was the expectation of most benefactors and administrations. As a result, even those centers with large amounts of initial funding and considerable administrative support are working to calibrate fiscal flows. The emphasis on making a profit reflects the priorities of many hospital administrators, as well as a newly formed group of philanthropists who provide seed money support to a small network of centers called the Bravewell Collaborative Clinical Network. This emphasis on profits creates dissonance with the philosophy of many practitioners and with their prior or ongoing experiences with sustained financial viability in a solo practice, direct fee-for-service environment.

Most centers must rely partially on private funding, in the form of either donations or patient payments. The majority of centers in our study have found that fund-raising is a permanent condition of their existence. In most cases, directors work with the hospital or university development office, which may often place its own restrictions on fund-raising and the availability of funds raised. Some directors have found the job of fund-raising encumbered by academic center policies that forbid them from tapping the same private donors as the hospital. Others have found donors for the center who would otherwise never have considered contributing to the hospital, only to then lose them to the larger hospital fund-raising program. One center negotiated an explicit policy regarding fund-raising and assignment of contributed funds with their parent organization.

The vast majority of outpatients at the centers we studied pay up front and out of pocket. In one center most of the cash flow comes from the overhead that clinicians charge patients. Although some patients have insurance coverage, reimbursements for CAM practitioners are low. As a result, only about half of the centers in our study accept insurance and even then not all plans. Those centers that are closely tied to their hospital's financial structure must accept whatever insurance the hospital accepts. Most commonly, these are managed care or preferred provider types of plans, which reimburse less than 75% of practitioners' charges. A few centers accept only Medicare, others only Medicaid, both of which reimburse at less than 75% of costs. Acceptance of insurance payments at some centers is seen as part of their commitment to providing access to the community at large, reflecting values of the parent organization when it is still controlled by a community-based board of trustees. A few practitioners have submitted grants to various agencies for funding for the indigents who visit their centers. A few centers leave to each practitioner the decision of whether to accept insurance. For the most part, even patients with insurance pay first and are then assisted if need be in their reimbursement procedures. Some of the inpatient services are covered by the hospital (sometimes through insurance) if approved by a physician.

How MDs charge both patients and third-party payers for their services at the centers varies. MDs who are both medical and clinical director generally bill insurers in some way if their patients are covered. One such director admitted she tries to bill for everything she does at the center insofar as her reimbursements are higher than those for practitioners. Another director indicated she often does not charge patients for consultations if they do not have insurance coverage.

None of the center directors in our study believes that insurance will expand in the near future, despite a recommendation to this effect by the White House Commission on Complementary and Alternative Health Policy.[130] This Clinton commission represents what is largely a lame duck effort because, despite efforts by Sen. Tom Harkin (D-Iowa), the work of the commission under the Clinton administration was so delayed that the report did not arrive until the Bush administration, which has shown little interest.

Nor are center directors putting much faith in the role of insurance in easing their financial problems, although all believe that expanded insurance coverage would enhance the legitimacy of CAM. They were unanimous in stating that, in a university hospital setting, patient payments alone are an insufficient source of funds to cover the costs of running a center. One reason lies in the nature of CAM work. It is more labor intensive and time consuming per patient than conventional medicine; the volume of services at IHCs is therefore much lower. Another reason is the high overhead, operational, and compliance costs of using high-tech hospital space for therapies that can be delivered in much less expensive spaces.

One additional source of funds is research grants, which are essential at academic centers, for the overhead they yield. Some directors told us that grants were their lifeline, funding large parts of their own salaries and those of other faculty at the center. Other directors, especially in centers that had not yet pursued research grants, expressed concern about growing pressure from university administrators to do so. How much overhead accrues to the centers varies, however, and is a source of tension for faculty who also have departmental appointments. Nevertheless, all of the center directors firmly believe that research-based publications, especially in mainstream medical journals, are an important source of legitimacy for CAM as well as for their IHC. Unfortunately, while always relatively underfunded, federal research funding for CAM is stagnating after 15 years of growth (Chapter 1).

A number of the centers operate on a year-to-year basis. One director confessed that "the hospital bails [the center] out at the end of the year because [it] can't balance [its] budget yet." Some directors revealed that their centers lose money for the hospital. One director indicated that the vice president of the hospital "just wants the center to not step on any toes and to break even." This director would like to "get out of having the same tax ID as the hospital, but the VP says it would just raise a red flag."

Accordingly, to balance their budgets and plan for the future, centers engage in additional activities. Classes in movement, art, and music therapies can realize more revenue per practitioner than do private sessions. One IHC holds retreats that combine learning and practice. In an effort to recruit more patients, centers engage in various kinds of community outreach, whether placing ads in local newspapers or giving talks and demonstrations either at the IHC or in local establishments. Brochures are generally distributed throughout the hospital and in selected community venues. The ability of some IHCs to engage in these activities is precluded by small size and insufficient personnel.

It would appear, then, that as they are presently structured, university hospital-based IHCs are not financially self-sustaining. Patient payments do not meet the bottom line; when private donations run out, new donors must be sought; and research funds require a supportive administrative and academic infrastructure. Although most directors in our study are optimistic about their future due to their supportive environments, some remain uncertain. Although many directors express the hope of eventual expansion, many acknowledge they would have problems increasing volume because they would need more space, staff, and so forth, all of which require more resources than they have or than will be made available.

A major problem for some of the financially-strained IHCs in our study is their university hospital base, with its burdensome overhead costs and bureaucratic regulations. Whether the university or the hospital affiliation or both is the more onerous varies to the extent that it is even clear. Accordingly, with the help of donors who cover initial start-up costs at the least, a few centers have begun to disengage financially and legally from their universities. Being separate entities enables them to control overhead costs and thereby achieve financial viability. They are or are planning to run the centers as independent facilities, contracting with practitioners on a salary, fee for service, or hourly basis, perhaps on a full-time status. Center directors who envision or already have such independence expect to maintain their faculty appointments and clinical privileges with the university hospital in order to treat inpatients and continue their research ties with faculty.

Compounding the vicissitudes of their own situations, the fate of IHCs everywhere is closely intertwined with the economic future both of CAM and of conventional medicine, as well as its relationship therewith. Many hospital boards and administrators in our study had presumed that CAM would be a cash cow, attracting clients who were willing to spend large sums of money on low-cost services. This expectation has not yet been met, which is not to say it may not in some way materialize. Many of the "wealthy well" are served in resort/spa settings.

There has not yet been sufficient study of the financial viability of IHCs that are not affiliated with either universities or hospitals, although there is hope everywhere that CAM can contribute to reduced expenditures on conventional medicine. However, while some studies support this hope, too few have been conducted and their investigations are limited, making generalizations difficult.[131] In searching for ways to survive financially, let alone prosper, center directors are learning from each other, and from the experiences of both those that are succeeding and those IHCs that have had to close for financial reasons.

Another large-scale consideration is the implication of tying centers into the mainstream hospital and health care system in the first place (Chapter 1). Many experts are predicting that the health care system is not financially viable beyond the early years of the next decade. For example, former U.S. Secretary of Health and Human Services (and governor of Wisconsin) Tommy Thompson has publicly stated that the current health care system can not continue in its present form and has established the

Center for Health Solutions in Washington, DC, to work toward alternatives. Integration of CAM services may be coming at just the wrong time to provide a financially viable alternative to a 20th century health care system that is not sustainable in the 21st century.

CONCLUSION

Although IHCs enjoy a special place in health care insofar as there are donors willing to fund the experiment they represent, they face specific and unique challenges in their struggle for financial viability. More research on how integrative medicine can save costs and generate revenues is sorely needed. This enterprise offers new opportunities for IHCs to forge links with researchers by providing investigative sites. Through such organizations as the Collaboration for Healthcare Renewal Foundation, some IHCs are joining providers, payers, insurers, educators, philanthropists, and others in working groups to discuss various issues, including cost-effectiveness. As studies mount, we may see integrative medicine emerge as one area of health care in which quality and cost are not contradictory.

CHAPTER 5

Getting Through the Door

Staffing and Credentialing Complementary Providers

CREDENTIALING AND STAFFING

Understanding credentialing is critical to staffing the integrative health care center. Credentialing, while readily understood for physicians and allied health providers (such as nurses, psychologists, and physical therapists), often challenges institutions seeking to integrate CAM practitioners such as chiropractors and acupuncturists. Yet, models of credentialing for CAM practitioners derive in large part from existing models within the conventional domain.

One of the critical differences, though, involves the presence (or absence) of clinical privileges. Physicians who are credentialed within a hospital typically receive such privileges, which include the ability to admit patients to the hospital and deliver clinical services to in-patients.[132] Such privileges also carry certain contractual rights, set forth in the institution's medical staff bylaws, as well as Fourteenth Amendment due process rights. These contractual and constitutional rights often make it difficult for the institution to terminate its employment relationship with the provider without certain rigorous, procedural protections.[133]

Most CAM practitioners in integrative health care centers presently lack authorization to treat inpatients, and in any event, lack the educational background and clinical training to admit patients to a hospital; clinical privileges, thus, may be unnecessary. Put another way, it is possible to credential CAM practitioners to deliver clinical services within an integrative health care center, without granting them clinical privileges or making them a member of the hospital's medical staff. This separation of credentialing from privileging has allowed some institutions to accept CAM professionals as providers of outpatient services, without having to battle for acceptance as part of the institution's medical staff.

Nonetheless, credentialing obstacles persist. Because of the historical antagonism between biomedical and CAM communities and the slow rate of medical acceptance for CAM therapies generally (as evidenced by the changing nomenclature), the effort to credential CAM practitioners—to allow them to deliver health care services within the institution—even apart from clinical privileges, can still generate controversy and difficulty. The following case studies give examples of these obstacles as well as sample strategies used to overcome institutional barriers.*

CASE STUDIES: PARADIGMS AND POLITICS

Most centers indicated that legal counsel was affiliated with the larger hospital but not present on a daily basis at the center; further, credentialing processes used for CAM practitioners were adapted from existing procedures within the hospital and negotiated with chairs of credentialing committees and other key personnel over a protracted period. Also, in most centers, to gain political buy-in within the institution, proponents of the integrative health care center brought together key players from the hospital, making the argument that doing so would help create quality assurance. But each center had different perspectives and stories of successes and failures. Our case studies show how attempts to create political buy-in were shaped in different institutions.

Case 5A: "Opportunity to Set Standards"

The medical director of one center reported that, in attempting to gain institutional support to bring CAM practitioners into the organization, his group presented the process of creating CAM credentialing standards to the medical board as an "opportunity to create a university-wide policy that will set standards, scope of practice, and make this more accessible to the university as a whole." The effort to present a win–win

---

*Notably, this chapter focuses on credentialing of CAM providers to deliver clinical services; credentialing conventional providers (including physicians and nurses) to offer CAM therapies typically involves efforts to educate department chiefs (and sometimes legal counsel) to include specified CAM therapies on the list of privileges available (with requisite training) to hospital staff. For example, recent years have seen the addition of mental health therapies such as biofeedback and hypnotherapy to privilege rosters for appropriately trained providers.

situation apparently succeeded: "We said we wanted to let them know what we're doing, and to bring consistency and standardization across the university—they saw this as a bonus." To implement their strategy, the medical director helped set up an ad hoc credentialing subcommittee of the executive medical board, consisting of key personnel assembled so as to create a political consensus (see Table 5.1).

The medical director reported that he brought supporting documentation to the committee and noted for his peers that other, respected institutions were engaged in similar efforts, some of which were problematic, and others that were easy to solve. The committee then worked on crafting a mock credentialing system based on documents the medical director had helped prepare.

These documents took advantage of resources from professional organizations and communities of practitioners. As an example, to credential yoga therapists within the health center, the medical director reported that he looked to

> what's out there—general national guidelines for the community, what's going on in other medical centers. I did a lot of sleuthing— went to all the schools on-line, figured out their teacher training and advanced courses, requirements, whether any do therapeutic yoga; found the Yoga Alliance, which has qualifications for registered yoga therapists; interviewed leaders in the field; came up with requirements and standards.

Again, the medical director's homework paid off in that his research ultimately was adopted by the institution: "The Medical Staff Office then put what I had written into a credentialing template," on the basis of which

---

TABLE 5.1   Key Personnel for Ad Hoc Credentialing Subcommittee of Hospital Executive Medical Board

- Medical director for the integrative health care center
- Director of finance and administration for the integrative health care center
- Chief medical officer for the medical center
- Office of the president—general counsel and assistant general counsel
- Committee on Interdisciplinary Practice (which is responsible for all allied health professionals)
- Medical staff office director
- Two chief medical officers for campus on which the integrative health care center is located
- Chair of the Credentialing Committee

---

providers were later credentialed and allowed to offer clinical services within the institution.

The director of risk management clarified:

> What we did . . . was decide the criteria for different practitioners, because it's not uniform within the state. For example, for massage therapists and yoga, we had to decide the number of years of clinical experience, hours of training we wanted them to have, what types of training. It's not uniform throughout the state. We demanded the highest level of credentialing and number of hours. We set the bar fairly high. I drafted applications for providers, based on the one for MDs and allied health providers—e.g., have you ever been subject to litigation, been subject to judgments, settled any claims, arising out of care you've provided. We have lists of privileges within certain divisions to perform certain activities. Not everyone within the department of medicine has the same privilege—some require monitoring or proctoring, some are highly specialized and require proof of competency. The Medical Staff Office does this, working with department chairs.

Case 5B: "It Was Easy Once the Scope Was Developed"

Another center director reported a different process, involving not only persuasion of stakeholders and study of existing credentialing schemes within the CAM professions, but also taking advantage of the comprehensive credentialing process within the larger health system, in which the integrative care clinic sits. That system is composed of several large hospitals and numerous smaller clinics, some affiliated with a university medical center. The health care system had set up a two-tiered credentialing process for its providers: (1) at the level of the health care system and (2) at the level of the entity (individual hospital or clinic).

At the level of the health care system, a committee was created to review and approve the scope of practice for different CAM practitioners, such as acupuncture (both inpatient and outpatient), Rolfing, and chiropractic. The committee did not credential or approve individual providers. Once scope of practice was developed at a system level, however, and then at the hospital level, the center was allowed to hire an individual provider (e.g., an acupuncturist) to deliver clinical services within that scope. Then followed a local review within the hospital in which the center sat of the scope of practice for that type of provider; the hospital committee could further narrow, but not broaden, the scope of practice authorized by the hospital system.

The director commented that this process made it feasible to bring providers to the institution with little additional effort, once the preliminary work was done at the higher levels: "We had three acupuncturists at the hospital, and it was easy to bring them on once the scope was developed [at the system level and then refined by the hospital]."

Case 5C: "That's Discriminatory; That's Racketeering"

In a third center, an acupuncturist who helped start the integrative health care center reported much internal controversy around credentialing CAM practitioners. In his own case, he was credentialed by the hospital to help treat inpatients and did so without institutional barriers for a period of time. But when physicians and administrators discovered he was using a fuller range of modalities within traditional Oriental medicine than simply the act of putting needles in a patient, the major department heads began to object, and became involved in trying to define what he could and could not do.

The acupuncturist explained:

> You have to meet with each department to allow you to practice that specialty. For example, you have to meet with orthopedists to practice on someone with knee pain. The departments wanted us to make sure conventional bases were covered, but the problem was the orthopedists and rheumatologists wouldn't talk to each other, because they compete with each other. They didn't want an acupuncturist to see the patient—they wanted to route the patient through this whole maze.

The acupuncturist also commented on the byzantine process of drafting standards for the providers: It "was like the NIH Consensus Panel [on Acupuncture]—let's see what it can help with; and what we can keep out." The process stagnated for many months, as major working groups could not come to agreement. A major reason for the discordance, in addition to internal disputes, was the fact of inadequate insurance coverage for CAM therapies. According to the acupuncturist, the mindset of some colleagues was, "If we can't bill insurance, then it [the therapy] doesn't fit our model." Another subgroup argued: "We have to wait until the state covers it in order to bring in acupuncture." These barriers, according to the acupuncturist, were difficult to surmount as they involved others' opinions about what steps had to come first. The acupuncturist criticized the "lack of integration within the allopathic model" and gave the following example:

> Suppose the patient comes in with knee pain. The orthopedist says, "Take 800 mg Motrin." The patient says it's better, but the orthopedist says, "It looks like arthritis. Go to the rheumatologist." The

rheumatologist says, "Take Methotrexate and Vioxx." The patient [does this and] says, "I'm not getting better, I want to see an acupuncturist." The rheumatologist says, "We'll send you to the endocrinologist to look at your immune system, [another specialist to look for] infectious disease, and then to a general practitioner; then to psychiatry, if that doesn't work. I can't write you a referral, because I want to figure out what this is not and rule things out. Then there's the nutritionist, physical therapy . . . eventually they get to the acupuncturist. Where's the patient? It takes 2–4 weeks to see each provider.

Yet another hurdle was the demand that the acupuncturist compile a list of medical conditions his treatments could address. According to the acupuncturist, this task raised issues of philosophical, cultural, and linguistic differences between the two professions (medicine and acupuncture). Indeed, the request was "impossible, because we [acupuncturists] handle illnesses from a totally different perspective. For example, they call it 'knee pain,' we look at balance." The acupuncturist complained that the credentialing committee was setting up a double standard, because physicians were credentialed by checking off what procedures they can and cannot perform without being asked to justify how they treat a given condition, whereas he was being asked to go into details of his treatment protocol. Further, the committee was essentially limiting his scope of practice to using needling to treat nausea from chemotherapy and radiation sickness (that is, the therapeutic use of acupuncture found effective by the NIH Consensus Panel). The acupuncturist remarked: "That's discriminatory; that's racketeering."

He also reported suggesting to peers that rather than requiring such lengthy, verbal justification, physicians should simply refer patients and look for improvement; thus, if the specialists had patients they could not cure, they should send those patients to him. This, he suggested, would not violate the obligation of nonmaleficence; he pointed out that patients with diagnoses such as chronic fatigue, fibromyalgia, and Epstein-Barr have diseases of unknown etiology, so that referring them for acupuncture could do no harm. To some extent, he reported, these arguments, while initially controversial, ultimately succeeded with many physicians, as "the relationship took over, and they let me see patients"—even though the credentialing standards had not been finalized.

Ultimately, as the institution gained more comfort with acupuncture, credentialing standards were developed. This was done in large part by appropriately modifying existing institutional standards for medical doctors. Part of this effort involved sorting out providers who were using the title *acupuncturist* illicitly. This required deciding which providers within the institution, who were offering some modality within the corpus of acupuncture and traditional Oriental medicine, would *no longer* be able to call themselves "acupuncturists:"

> I worked with the chair of the credentialing committee. . . . There were some MDs [from different countries] practicing acupuncture in the hospital who lacked U.S. credentials; [for example,] nurses practicing auricular therapy (as in detoxification programs) who called themselves 'acupuncturists.' I had to sort out that these providers would *not* have the acupuncture credential.

In the end, though, the acupuncturist reported, despite the previously noted successes, the process never came to fruition. Other institutional difficulties—in particular, a severe financial crisis within the larger institution—overshadowed the effort to create a financially sustainable, integrative care clinic. Even if the clinic itself was financially viable, the overarching financial woes of the larger institutions made the clinic financially untenable. This situation may serve as a warning for the general issue of trying to make integrative medicine practice financially viable within a health care system that is not sustainable.

This latter observation was, in fact, echoed in several other institutions; as one center's director put it, "[we had] little to no struggle with credentialing. But the infrastructure and financial issues were so profound that we decided to close the clinic." This interviewee also reported that the "biggest challenge" the center faced was the process of getting third-party reimbursement for CAM services: "As we successfully obtained contracts with third-party payers, we were bound to financial terms that the health system and hospital set (for example, with Blue Cross). So the more patients we saw, the more money we lost. We were tied to contracts of the health system." She summarized "the lesson" as follows: "It's important to have either freedom from the health center to negotiate contracts, or operate on a cash basis." The risk manager at another center reported as the center's biggest challenge:

> trying to convince at least the older generation of physicians (of) the benefits of alternative therapies and that they can help people and that it's something the community is interested in. There's a certain amount of skepticism in a certain physician age population about . . . whether these therapies are really helping patients or just have a placebo effect.

Case 5D: "Fast Track"

In a fourth center, to gain institutional buy-in, the administrator initially approached the hospital's credentialing committee and the credentialing body for allied health professionals. The administrator found that, in general, the committees "didn't know what to do with" the idea of credentialing licensed acupuncturists to deliver clinical services, and with allowing physician assistants and registered nurses to use designated CAM therapies. The committees began working to create standards regarding such matters as who could supervise the acupuncturists and what criteria would be necessary in terms of providers' clinical training and experience. The process of developing these [standards] took an entire year; this, however, was considered a fast track that was facilitated because an affiliated institution had already started working on the forms and the credentialing process for acupuncturists.

During this process, it was easier to establish standards and processes to credential massage therapists than acupuncturists. Because massage therapists were not under the auspices of medical staff credentialing and were not considered allied health professionals, they could be hired within the institution as employees. In other words, the massage therapists probably were credentialed through the human resources department, in a more abbreviated process, rather than through the committee that credentialed allied health professionals. Such a pathway has the benefit of economy and efficiency, although it arguably is not as thorough as moving providers through the approval of a hospital committee.

Case 5E: "They Know I'm Legit"

The prior examples are ones in which dedicated individuals sought to persuade relevant committees to accept or include CAM practitioners such as acupuncturists and massage therapists within the institution. A fifth center emerged out of an extended public-relations campaign for holistic therapies that took the form of years of educational programs within the institution around topics in integrative care, including: "mindfulness meditation, Qi Gong, Tai Chi, other movement and self-care practices." These course offerings recurred in multiple affiliated hospitals over years, and thus provided an opportunity to expose clinicians to a variety of unfamiliar therapies and practices.

According to the center's medical director, this long-standing focus on research and education regarding CAM therapies made the hospital administrators more receptive to CAM therapies, and particularly when, one day, the institution received a large donation from a patient with a mandate to try to find a model for integrative care. Following the donation, a task force was created at the medical center that included administrative and clinical leaders. Notably, this group included "the two major nay-sayers, healthy skeptics—chiefs of medicine and psychiatry." The inclusion of skeptics and their subsequent conversion to a position of

acceptance, or at least tolerance, for the proposed idea of integrati
was critical to the center's success. The medical director reported:

> I'm a political animal and chaired the department of . . . , have been
> here a long time, know everybody. They know I'm legit; I'm not the
> Birkenstock, tie-dyed guy who worked in the emergency room.

The director's experience and credibility within the hospital apparently
helped generate consensus, as did his decision to include adversaries as
well as allies:

> We started with a significant task force and also got legal counsel
> on board. This was 5–6 years ago and nobody really knew what the
> hell to do. We staffed it with board-certified MDs who had member-
> ship in [the right] departments. [The] MDs on [our] clinical staff—
> each a member of a specialty department within the hospital—are
> credentialed through the Medical Staff Office, which has its own
> core competencies the provider must demonstrate (for example in
> acupuncture); I sign off, and then the chief of medicine does.

The director concluded:

> We've played the game pretty well so we have few legal and other
> institutional issues. . . . When CAM came along and got popular, it
> was easy to ground our work. We had no money, lots of skepti-
> cism, space issues, many challenges.

In short, through astute maneuvering and consensus-building, the center
opened and apparently began to flourish.

Case 5F: "What I Need Is More Physicians Like Me"

In one institution, credentialing guidelines already existed for licensed
acupuncturists, approved through the hospital's medical staff office. Yet,
for financial reasons, an acupuncturist was never hired:

> Even though they approved the credentialing guidelines, there is a
> budget crunch, and people see this as a luxury. They know by now
> that this center and kind of treatment is not a moneymaker. If they
> would see it as a marketing tool for the institution as a whole, it
> may become more attractive in the future.

In part as a result of this experience, the medical director stated:

> My vision is not to add CAM practitioners here—I'm happy collab-
> orating with them in the community. What I need is more physicians

like me, because there's a huge demand for physicians who practice integrative medicine. I can't satisfy the demand and as well would enjoy colleagues who share ideas. A mind–body therapist and someone who is osteopathically trained would be ideal.

The medical director also expressed antipathy toward chiropractors as opposed to medically trained osteopathic counterparts: "Some chiropractors just do adjustments and don't understand body functioning the way osteopaths do (e.g., understand soft tissue, exercises, positions, postures)." An added point was that the American Holistic Medical Association and the American Board of Holistic Medicine now certifies holistic physicians, a practice that may add to the position that MDs constitute valuable representatives for CAM therapies within an integrative care team.

Case 5G: "Tell Us About Complications"

The director of risk management for a large, academic medical center with multiple, affiliated hospitals had little to say about credentialing, except that "strong credentialing is important" to maintaining the integrity of the integrative care clinical team, as well as to minimizing potential liability exposure. This individual also noted the challenge in training CAM practitioners regarding the credentialing and quality assurance requirements of a conventional care center:

> They have to tell us about complications when they occur; some practitioners are foreign and we have to educate them regarding reporting, documentation, and dealing with complications.

Case 5H: Finding Mechanisms, Avoiding Lawsuits

The Senior VP we interviewed indicated they made "case-by-case decisions as to which providers to include and which modalities to offer." Because the center is "evidence-based, has ties in traditional research, and does not exclude conventional medicine from the therapeutic armamentarium," it may be possible to include CAM therapies that "do no harm," even if potential benefit is "still up to question." The other concern is that in hospitals with oversight by bodies such as Department of Health and the Joint Commission on Accreditation of Healthcare Organizations (JCAHO):

> There is a lot of regulatory scrutiny, peer pressure, and peer review by medical staff as a whole, Medical Executive Committee, and

departmental leadership, so there is a tighter control over what physicians are allowed to do or what is considered appropriate. In a private physician's office, doctors stretch the envelope (although this can become a concern to the state medical board, since that is the only oversight).

The Senior VP gave an example of the competing concerns. Apparently a chiropractor asked for privileges and membership in the medical staff. The medical staff bylaws did not have a mechanism to allow this. In a similar case within the state, the chiropractor sued the hospital. Following the court's analysis, the senior VP indicated how the hospital would make a decision about the chiropractor's request:

> [First] we would say: is there a patient care need (because our mission is to meet the community's needs), a demand by our patients, physicians; is it appropriate for us? [Next we would] weigh the administrative burdens of bylaws amendments; creating a credentialing process for a new type of provider; peer review; quality oversight; [and ask,] is there an increased [risk of] medical malpractice?

The VP concluded by noting that in an acute care hospital, with an average length of stay of 5 days, resources are limited; such resource limitations would be taken into account in addressing the chiropractor's request.

Case 5I: "All MDs and Nurses Right Now"

One center's administrator noted that there were "no credentialing issues to date since we're all MDs and nurses right now." However, the research director for this new clinical center indicated:

> One way to handle credentialing is that we find people already credentialed at the institution—e.g., nurse practitioner, dietician—who do something else.

In responding to a question about contact with the hospital's legal counsel, the interviewee also noted that "the lawyer has been supportive and creative in figuring out how to solve potential problems."

Case 5J: "One of the Attorneys. . . ."

At one institution, the credentialing process itself was not difficult; it involved such tasks as "checking competencies—we covered basic things like education and training." But institutional politics presented major hurdles.

The key issues involved scope of practice, but the center's leaders "tried to be congruent with state laws [regarding] supervision and referrals." The founders "knew ahead of time these would be issues," and that the MDs within the hospital "were afraid of credentialing acupuncturists."

In response, the center set up policy such that if the patient was neither referred to the center by an MD, nor had an MD on file within the hospital system, then that patient would need to see the center's medical director. They also arrange for supervised history-taking and physicals—for example, the MD-acupuncturist would supervise the technical skills of the non-MD acupuncturist. Thus, for "every new acupuncture patient, the medical director reviews the case notes or talks directly to the acupuncturist and writes an addendum for the medical charts." This risk management tool doubled as an effort to reassure those in the hospital responsible for setting up a credentialing program for CAM practitioners. The policy added that the center does not offer primary care, but rather coordinates with the patient's primary care doctor. The administrator also noted that "some patients are more open to CAM therapies, such as acupuncture, once a physician recommends them."

Despite these protections, "one of the attorneys got a little anal about acupuncture." Initially, the plan was to hire CAM practitioners under job descriptions—to have them credentialed but not given medical staff privileges.

> Because one of the lawyers was nervous about this, we had to go through our medical staff president and the executive committee to get input regarding acupuncture. They were supportive but wanted to cover themselves. There was also a control issue in that our program does not report to ambulatory care and emergency services; we are not lumped in with all the other outpatient clinics. So the person who thought he would oversee us found out someone else in the hospital had jurisdiction. We put together a white paper and politicked. Ultimately, legal counsel told us we probably didn't have to jump all these hoops. What we provided was so thorough and overwhelming that they have few questions. Also, we had already hired the practitioners before getting approval.

This thorough homework and the fait accompli helped the center accomplish its objectives. Another factor was that the current hospital board was "younger, forward thinking, [more] open-minded than what we had a year ago; we probably would not have gotten this approved a year or so ago." The medical director and administrator also were able to help an MD-acupuncturist get privileged within the hospital, and thus support the credentialing process for the non-MD acupuncturist.

The interviewee noted that the "next hurdle" for the program is chiropractic. Interdepartmental outreach was perceived as key to this effort, and so was good fortune:

> We're talking to neurosurgery, neurology, orthopedics and asking them to stand up at the medical board and speak for us. We keep having changes in department chairs that help us—timing is everything.

Case 5K: "Creating Something New and Different"

One center responded that it uses "only state-licensed therapists, including massage therapists." If the center wishes to offer a therapy at the edge of what is medically acceptable, it will have the therapy provided by a licensed practitioner within the scope of practice. For example, there are three different practitioners who can offer reflexology: the nurse, the massage therapist, and the physical therapist. Each practitioner must be "nationally certified if such certification exists" for that particular modality. In addition, as part of its credentialing scheme, the center requires that applicants have a significant level of practice experience (preferably at least 5 years).

This center experienced considerable "hurdles or more like challenges: we were creating something new and different" by creating integration.

> When we first hired our acupuncturist, the hospital did not want the MD-acupuncturist to be part of the appointed staff, but to be hired as an acupuncturist-employee. As the hospital grew more comfortable with us, we were able to hire experienced, non-MD, licensed acupuncturists without necessarily having MD-acupuncturists.

Even having hired the non-MD acupuncturist, the institution disallows use of moxa, "because it involves setting something on fire," and disallows cupping, because it "involves bruising." The concern appears to be as much the potentially negative political impact of these therapies as their safety aspects. The director noted:

> There are many aspects of CAM that we have nothing to do with; we only allow therapies if they're rational and we have data.

But even then, the director stated, "we know what's accepted and what's appropriate in our institutional setting." This center has excluded modalities such as homeopathy, craniosacral therapy, Native American healing ("although we do some chanting occasionally"), crystal healing, and energy therapies.

One of the unusual therapies being offered is music therapy. The center found that in planning a clinical trial, creating the protocol posed difficulties, because the center was required to have the university system's general counsel to "rule on intellectual property issues before we can even get started" (e.g., downloading music clips from the Web based on what the patient chooses). The center, it turns out, "received a favorable ruling," based on several factor including obtaining clearance to purchase subscriptions to the Web sites (the researchers had to read all the terms on-line), use of "a specific formula for how patients will choose the music based on the patient's mood and need/desire to alter the mood therapeutically with combinations of rhythm and length of music," and a commitment to collect and destroy the CDs used, once the study ends.

Case 5L: "We Haven't Tried to Do Anything Controversial"

One center noted that it "quickly" developed procedures and guidelines for approving certain educational or self-care programs (such as mind–body, nutrition, and yoga) that could be offered to patients. The center facilitated this process by linking the clinician offering the program with a faculty mentor (such as a medical doctor or a mental health professional, e.g., psychologist, social worker) to be sure the sponsor understood the issues. The medical director noted:

> We haven't tried to do anything controversial in clinical delivery;
> we have focused on mind–body therapies.

This particular center has two part-time massage therapists on staff and is hiring a full-time acupuncturist. For these providers, credentialing "was not much of an issue, because both occupations have solid licensure processes." Further, the center ensures that patients receive "an informal consultation" from the medical director and that this will become more formalized in the future. The larger challenge involved setting up an appropriate fee structure, because the center does not bill insurance for services offered by these providers.

The theme of "stringent . . . credential review" was repeated across several centers. As one center leader explained, "a lot of well-meaning people wanted to bring their programs to us, but many lacked the experience or organization to do so." This center offers many educational and self-care programs to patients—involving numerous outside contractors who come for a brief period to offer such programs—and therefore uses a variety of steps to screen applicants.

> The first is a simple, two-page form that is our first-line: who will
> facilitate it, what are the goals, what goes on in a simple session,

who is the audience, what are the logistics. We weed some people out because they realize this is a real process and they may not be sufficiently developed. For the ones who come through, we have a committee made of individuals who have experience related to the content of the program meet with the applicant (for example, someone from physical and rehabilitation medicine will meet with movement therapists). We ask how they'll adapt their program to our population, what is their experience with our population, and what's in it for them. That makes them reflect; we also weed out those simply looking for referrals or to sell a product. We then gather all their certificates of training, references; we speak with their clients (within constraints of confidentiality). They do a demonstration for us—perhaps a class for our staff. If we're still unsure, we'll have our quality assurance advisor sit in on at least six sessions to provide oversight and feedback.

The interviewee also explained how the center manages scope of practice in such a complex program involving more than a hundred different practitioners. If a practitioner desires to offer a service outside her typical expertise (for example, a senior nurse who offers aromatherapy), the center first has the provider offer that service on a volunteer basis for several years, gauging safety and patient need. Thus, "only now are we developing budgets for activities such as Tibetan meditation, Qi Gong, and a Reiki master."

ISSUES INVOLVING SCOPE OF PRACTICE BOUNDARIES

The decision to allow a given CAM practitioner (or group of practitioners) to deliver clinical services within the institution is a starting point. As some of the case studies have alluded, an equally controversial issue involves determining the acceptable parameters of a provider's practice. While the fact of CAM practitioner licensure varies by state (for example, naturopathic physicians are licensed in less than a quarter of the states),[134] the legal scope of practice authorized to CAM practitioners by licensing laws also varies by state.[135] For example, licensed chiropractors can offer nutritional advice in some states but not others; licensed acupuncturists can recommend Chinese herbs in some states but not others; and naturopathic physicians can, in some states, prescribe over-the-counter medications and certain prescription drugs or, with appropriate training, facilitate natural childbirth.[136]

Legal scope of practice boundaries have a legitimate purpose: they "aim to ensure that providers offer services according to their skill and training and do not induce overreliance by patients on nonmedical therapies for a cure."[137] However, as discussed in Chapter 2, scope of practice boundaries also tend to carve the patient into parts, assigning, for example, the muscles to massage therapists, the emotions to psychologists, and the spine to chiropractors.[138]

Significant disputes have arisen as to whether CAM practitioners have exceeded their scope of practice, despite legislative authorization that may have appeared unambiguous. For example, in *Stockwell v. Washington State Chiropractic Disciplinary Board*,[139] a chiropractor challenged a disciplinary action based on selling and dispensing vitamins to patients. The chiropractor argued that his practices were within Washington's chiropractic licensing statute, which authorized chiropractors to provide "dietary advice" to their patients. The court, upholding the board's decision to discipline the chiropractor, held that mere advice differed from prescribing vitamins,[140] but it did not draw any formal, rational distinction between "advice" and "prescription."

CAM practitioners who exceed their legislatively authorized scope of practice may not only be disciplined by their own boards, but also prosecuted for unauthorized practice of "medicine."[141] But if CAM practitioners deliver services within scope of practice boundaries, such services may be deemed by a health care institution to lack sufficient proof of safety or efficacy, and thereby to be suspect. Alternatively, if the provider's services have a mechanism that is unknown (or are explained by theories that are considered implausible, such as notions of yin and yang in acupuncture or theories of subluxation in chiropractic), the institution may be reluctant to offer such services. Thus, one of the controversial arenas in credentialing involves the decision to limit providers' scope of practice more tightly than their authorization under the relevant licensing statute and accompanying administrative regulations and cases, if any.

Some centers are more lenient than others in this regard. For example, one interviewee noted:

> As medical director I meet with the providers on an annual basis, go over scope of practice issues, make sure they take courses to update their scope.

This center allows most CAM practitioners to practice to the fullest extent of their statutory authorization, even if the therapy (e.g., use of essential oils) has little, if any, support in the medical literature and thereby might be regarded as fringe:

> For example, with chiropractic, the provider uses essential oils; I go over the training required for her to do this. There are no standards for this practice, but there are courses dealing with toxicity, etc.

This medical director was asked to explain how the decision to allow such a therapy could be justified and how the director felt comfortable allowing such a therapy. The director responded:

> I have a postdoctoral fellowship that informs me. There are always "new" therapies that are in the institutional setting, and the fellowship helped me to do evidence-based research and discussion with peers to establish a standard for how to do this. The Consortium [of Academic Health Centers in Integrative Medicine] also will help in the future: Institutions could work together and come up with standards of practice for say, energy healing . . . [and how] to standardize herbal therapies and other treatments.

By way of comparison, another center director reported that one or more of its CAM practitioners had to accept the narrower practice boundaries imposed by the institution. It is not clear whether the decision was based on medical evidence or on the historic animus between the professions. Thus:

> A political nuance was that for chiropractic . . . [the credentialing committee] approved a narrower scope of practice than many chiropractors would find desirable, but it worked within the health system.

Like the initial decision to credential CAM practitioners, the decision to allow scope of practice boundaries to the fullest extent authorized by law, or to further narrow institutional scope, remains a controversial adaptation within each institution, with local politics affecting the results.[142]

OTHER MAJOR CHALLENGES

Centers used a range of credentialing mechanisms, from hospital privileging for medical doctors using CAM therapies to relying on the human resources department for many of the CAM practitioners. Thus, as one center has reported:

> Some CAM practitioners were credentialed through a medical staff review committee, but many we hired directly through HR. That worked well for massage therapists (because we had a job description for massage through physical therapy); nurses (healing touch); psychologists (already had a mechanism). A third track was hiring MDs. At one time we had three MDs. This was similar to hospital privileging.

Regarding other major challenges concerning credentialing, the medical director of one center reported:

> The various providers report to me. We are reviewed by JCAHO; we survey the charts for quality assurance. We do due diligence on them in the credentialing phase; interview peers; have a certain number of years required.

One question that the interviewees were not asked was the extent to which credentialing, including the process of obtaining political buy-in within the institution, resulted in a violation (real or perceived) of the mission, vision, or mandate of integrative care.[143] Rather, the interviews focused on the nitty-gritty details of how the interviewees moved their agendas through the system. Only one center director commented on the importance of mission in every facet of the center's operation. This interviewee volunteered detailed information about the center's philosophy and the way the aesthetic of the physical space was created to reflect that philosophy:

> We have a full-size 30-diameter labyrinth at the entrance. We remodeled the chapel in the main acute care hospital in a very pastoral motif (trees, water, nice lighting) to make it felt here. Integrative medicine really lives here. This is a large medical staff in a highly competitive market—managed care, etc. Lots of docs are depressed in the hospitals—are under it, economically. Our purpose in getting the clinic going was truly to complement their practice, and we honor their wish to spend more time with patients if they can afford it. We fund-raise a lot of money for scholarship and to support care (free; discounted) for those who cannot afford it, but the truth is we're doing fee-for-service medicine. So we do classes to support health-related change in people, teach in neighborhood centers.[144]

In short, although mission/vision were not necessarily perceived as having to be sacrificed for the sake of political achievement within the institution, few interviewees actively mentioned an emphasis on putting mission and vision in the foreground.

MODEL STRATEGIES FOR CREDENTIALING

Our interviews focused not only on the mechanics of credentialing, but also on the process of getting the institution to agree to credential CAM practitioners and therapies. Common strategies among interviewees included the following.

Increase Institutional Buy-In

Prior to attempting to credential CAM practitioners within the institution, a series of initiatives were aimed to bridge cultural consensus around the safety and efficacy of CAM therapy. Some of the substrategies to enhance buy-in included the following:

- Conduct several years of educational programs within the institution around practices such as mindfulness meditation, Qi Gong, Tai Chi, and other movement and self-care practices.
- Increase buy-in from hospital administration by adding medical doctors familiar with integrative care. As suggested, some centers opted out of including CAM practitioners and styled their integrative care efforts as having physicians (or nurses and other conventional providers) integrate CAM therapies, while referring out to selected CAM practitioners. Others included CAM practitioners, but weighted their personnel toward physicians.
- Work on interdepartmental outreach. Center leaders worked on departmental outreach to gain buy-in around credentialing, seeking supportive faculty members to sponsor educational patient programs and arguing that significant patient demand made allocation of sufficient resources a necessity.
- Include key institutional players (including skeptics and critics). To gain political buy-in within the institution, proponents of the integrative health care center brought together key players from the hospital, aiming to generate consensus by emphasizing the need for rigorous quality assurance and standardization across affiliated institutions.
- Balance patient demand against administrative and resource burden of adding CAM practitioners. By styling credentialing toward mechanisms used for conventional providers, centers were able to minimize the notion of doing something "new and different"—breaking boundaries—and better able to cohere novel efforts with what the institution had previously known and accepted.
- Focus on or de-emphasize CAM mission and vision. Centers varied on the extent to which they highlighted or softened the stated focus on a mission or vision involving integrative care.[145]

Adapt Credentialing Procedures for Allied Health Professionals

Credentialing policies for CAM practitioners were adapted from existing procedures within the hospital for allied health providers and negotiated with chairs of credentialing committees, department heads (including major skeptics and critics), and other key personnel over a protracted period. This process was easier when specific providers (e.g., acupuncturists) were already delivering clinical services within the governing institution or affiliated hospital.

Review Pertinent National Professional Standards

To adapt such standards, proponents looked to general, national guidelines for the profession in question (e.g., yoga therapy), including educational and testing requirements.

Rely, Where Possible, on Human Resources Mechanism

Depending on the institution, providers who were not under the auspices of medical staff credentialing, and were not considered allied health professionals, could be hired as employees (e.g., through the human resources department).

Carefully Negotiate Authorized Scope of Practice

Center leaders followed the "path of least resistance" by having providers already credentialed to deliver conventional therapies at the institution simply add CAM therapies within their scope of practice. Thus, it likely would be easier within the institution to have a nurse perform therapeutic touch than to hire an unlicensed provider to do so. As one medical director observed:

> We may have to have dual-degreed practitioners, such as a PA-Lac or ND-MD. The MD is the only one that bills; the CAM practitioners are students at CAM colleges who participate in the intake and write up a treatment plan and then e-mail it to the MD who refers the patients out. Each provider talks to the patient about their area. In a few years when the administration changes we'll have CAM practitioners on full-time.

Centers hiring CAM practitioners were not obligated to make such providers members of the medical staff, with staff privileges, but rather could use credentialing standards to ensure competence and then delineate what the providers could or could not do within the institution. Many centers chose to eliminate controversial modalities from a given provider's institutionally allowed scope of practice—for example, in a number of centers, acupuncturists could not recommend Chinese herbs;

similarly, in one center, massage was allowed for inpatients but limited to light touch. Others limited their clinical team to physicians (e.g., incorporating nutrition and mind–body therapies) to reduce controversy within the institution.

Educate Providers Toward Risk Management

Center leaders were able to move forward credentialing efforts within the institution by showing hospital administration that mechanisms were in place to educate CAM practitioners regarding documentation, reporting requirements, and other risk management procedures standard to hospital outpatient practice. In some cases, physician supervision was necessary to ensure that CAM practitioners did not exceed their scope of practice. Once again, a major premise of integrative care involves not abandoning conventional monitoring, diagnosis, and referral back to the patient's primary care when medically necessary.

While these ad hoc strategies appear to have been useful, no true consensus has emerged among hospitals generally as to which CAM practitioners to select from among the enormous variety available; how best to adopt existing institutional mechanisms; and how to integrate CAM providers more seamlessly into preventive care and medical treatment overall. Thus, a 2005 study of credentialing practices in 19 hospitals with integrative care centers revealed that "institutions had no consistent approaches to provider mix and authority within the integrative care team," and that hospitals "are using heterogeneous approaches to address licensure/credentialing/scope of practice, malpractice liability, and dietary supplement use in developing models of integrative care."[146] Similarly, the randomized survey mentioned earlier of 39 academic medical centers with respect to their CAM practices revealed that "few academic medical centers have sufficiently integrated CAM services into conventional care by developing consensus written policies governing credentialing" (as well as regarding malpractice liability and dietary supplement use).[147] The 2004 study of 33 academic medical centers mentioned earlier similarly concurred: "State licensure requirements for CAM providers appear to not be well understood. Most commonly CAM professionals do not receive full medical staff credentials."[148]

As a coda to the complex conversation regarding credentialing, bringing CAM providers into mainstream medical settings can be a mixed blessing, both for the providers and for the quality of CAM services they provide:

As a generalization, CAM providers both want the legitimacy of integration within an academic medical center, and feel constrained by institutional credentialing processes, scope of practice limitations, and other constraints. Credentialing poses a dark side in terms of increased con-striction of practice freedom. The flip side of this dynamic is that, from our study, many institutional champions of integrative care centers who are licensed medical directors or other conventional providers both respect principles of evidence-based medicine yet also appreciate the unsolved mysteries of Reiki, therapeutic touch, and other forms of subtle energy, while playing the evidence-based card to gain institutional legitimacy.[149]

CHAPTER 6

Staying Afloat

Minimizing Potential
Liability Exposure

MANAGING INDIVIDUAL LIABILITY RISK

The definition of malpractice given in chapter 3 is critical to understanding liability management: negligence involves practicing below the standard of care, which injures the patient. Standards of care vary by profession, for example, medicine, nursing, chiropractic, acupuncture. Thus, CAM providers who offer therapies that the profession itself considers unsafe or marginally effective may be courting liability.

The reverse statement is that therapies should be supported by reasonable evidence of safety and efficacy. A CAM treatment supported by such evidence is probably within the standard of care. In such a case, the medical expert for a physician defending against a medical malpractice charge would have ample basis for testifying that the CAM therapy chosen was within accepted clinical practice. Furthermore, the defendant's choice of such therapy likely would appear not to create an unreasonable danger to the patient. In short, understanding the availability of evidence regarding safety and efficacy provides a good map to potential liability.

One can think of a grid of clinical risk, with the x-axis indicating safety and the y-axis, efficacy. As shown in Figure 6.1, four quadrants indicate whether the medical evidence variously supports safety or efficacy, or is inconclusive regarding either.[150] This chart provides a working framework particularly for physicians contemplating how to advise patients concerning inclusion (or discontinuance) of CAM therapies in an integrative care regimen. In quadrant A, the therapy by definition is unlikely

B. Supports safety, but evidence regarding efficacy is inconclusive.	A. Supports safety and efficacy.
D. Indicates either serious risk or inefficacy.	C. Supports efficacy, but evidence regarding safety is inconclusive.

FIGURE 6.1   A clinical risk grid.

to cause injury and probably falls within the standard of care; its use therefore probably does *not* generate malpractice liability. In quadrant D, the therapy by definition is likely to cause injury or to fall below the standard of care; its use therefore probably *does* generate liability.

Most CAM therapies are likely to fall within quadrants B and C, in which either safety or efficacy concerns make the provider conceivably liable. Safety probably trumps efficacy, however, in that if a therapy is relatively safe, but the evidence regarding its efficacy is inconclusive, in general it would be more difficult to show that the therapy's use caused the patient injury (assuming an ineffective CAM therapy was not substituted for a conventional therapy deemed safe and effective). However, if evidence regarding safety is inconclusive and a patient is injured, it might be easier to assign the cause of the injury to the CAM therapy.[151]

A helpful way to help manage liability exposure is to determine the clinical risk level, using the grid in Figure 6.1. Whether the therapy falls within regions A, B, C, or D, a clinician respectively should (A) recommend and continue to monitor; (B) accept use, caution the patient, and monitor effectiveness; (C) accept use, caution the patient, and monitor safety; and (D) avoid and actively discourage patient use.[152] This framework is being used satisfactorily in a variety of settings, including specialties such as oncology[153] and cardiology.[154] Somewhat analogous models have also been used in pediatrics.[155] The clinician should realize, however, that as medical evidence changes, therapies can shift from one quadrant to another.

In addition, the clinician can help manage potential liability by (1) including a back-up file of the literature supporting the therapeutic choice and keeping clear notes in the medical record; (2) engaging the patient in a clear discussion of risks and benefits regarding the therapy, and if feasible, obtaining the patient's written, express agreement to use the treatment; and (3) continuing to monitor conventionally, and intervene conventionally when medically necessary.[156]

As an example, if the clinician recommends an herb, the clinician should, at a minimum, be certain there is no documented serious risk or proven inefficacy; document the choice of herb and rationale for this choice; and document any discussion regarding therapeutic dose, and any discussion with the patient concerning potential herb–drug interactions and other adverse effects or other therapeutic risks.

If the conventional caregiver is referring to (or comanaging the patient with) a CAM practitioner, a number of similar strategies are suggested. First, it probably will be helpful to know whether the CAM practitioner is using therapies that fall within an acceptable spectrum of risk in the grid. To the extent therapies fall in quadrant D, this is a red flag suggesting that referral may be inappropriate, while greater judgment is called for therapies in quadrants B and C.

Put another way, one should ask: "Is there evidence from the medical literature to suggest that the therapies a patient will receive as a result of the referral will offer no benefit or will subject the patient to unreasonable risks?"[157] If the answer is yes, the referral may be inadvisable, as it could potentially subject the referring provider to an undesirable level of liability risk.

In addition, at a minimum, the clinician should review (or ask legal counsel to review) the licensing statute for that CAM practitioner and get a good feel for what services the provider can and cannot provide, and inquire of any relevant licensing or regulatory body regarding the provider's history of malpractice litigation or disciplinary action.[158] It may also be helpful to review one's own malpractice insurance policy and make appropriate inquiries to the carrier—and get answers in writing, if possible—as to whether use of CAM therapies or referrals will be covered or subject to specific exclusions.

MANAGING INSTITUTIONAL LIABILITY RISK

As mentioned in chapter 3, in the conventional domain, direct negligence can include failure to supervise providers (as suggested in the earlier hypothetical), and, as well, failure to take sufficient quality assurance measures to ensure that providers within the institution are reasonably competent. Again, this should translate into the CAM domain. Institutions should ensure that providers who require supervision under state law indeed have the requisite supervision. Institutions also have a duty to take reasonable steps to ensure patient safety and well-being, using methods additional to ensuring appropriate supervision of providers; the duty includes maintaining safe and adequate facilities and equipment, and implementing rules and policies to ensure quality care.[159]

In the integrative care setting, regular team meetings may help ensure that conventional and CAM practitioners can share a common language and sufficiently communicate about different diagnostic and therapeutic techniques so that the patient is receiving due care. Further, the medical director or hospital administrator should ensure that whatever the system for patient flow, patients do receive conventional diagnostic monitoring and care as necessary.

Vicarious liability may be more difficult to manage, and indeed, vicarious liability concerns form an important obstacle to establishing integrative care within conventional medical settings. The legal landscape is ambiguous and underdeveloped at best, allowing fears and perceptions around malpractice liability issues to cloud institutional decision making. While fear of potential liability should not paralyze efforts to create integrative care, concern for potential liability requires implementing quality assurance and other procedures as suggested previously.

The combination of potential direct and vicarious liability imposes a legal catch-22 on health care institutions integrating CAM therapies: To the extent the institution loosens supervisory control over CAM practitioners in an effort to reduce the risk of vicarious liability, the organization thereby increases the risk of direct liability for negligent acts by those providers.[160] However, to the extent the institution increases supervisory control over CAM practitioners in an effort to reduce the risk of direct liability, the more it increases the risk of vicarious liability under an agency theory. Notably, where the negligent CAM provider is an employee, courts may impose vicarious liability under an agency theory irrespective of measures taken to control the provider's quality of care. Either way, the institution finds itself facing potential malpractice liability exposure for the negligent acts of CAM practitioners under its auspices.

One way to avoid such scenarios is to have strong credentialing criteria in place to ensure that providers are qualified and highly competent. Another is to determine what modalities, within a given CAM profession, present excessive risk, and impose institutional limitations on the provider's legislatively authorized scope of practice. The latter may be controversial if, for example, the scope of practice includes modalities (such as herbal therapy by acupuncturists) that are intrinsic to the profession yet not readily understood by physicians or that are widely used within the profession yet presently lacking in satisfactory mechanistic explanations.

A third liability management strategy is as suggested previously, to have policies and procedures to help ensure safety. For example, an institution may have a policy to ensure disposal of used acupuncture needles as a potential biohazard. Presumably, CAM practitioners, if hired as employees, will be bound to the many administrative and other policies and procedures of the hospital. This may include such simple public health measures as, for example, washing hands between clients, and a variety of other requirements for hospital clinicians and employees. The health care institution may need to implement some of these measures by written agreement with CAM practitioners who remain independent contractors. Simply denying patients the ability to access CAM therapies offers no easy solutions.[161] Rather, careful considerations of legal as well as economic issues can help health care institutions with the strategic planning necessary to ensure viable integration of CAM therapies and practitioners.[162]

TEAM PROCESSES—HANDLING CONFLICT

No consensus presently exists regarding ways to integrate perspectives from biomedical and multiple CAM disciplines in the art of diagnosis and treatment. Even within the domain of conventional care, questions have arisen concerning ways that health care providers such as social workers in hospice can successfully collaborate with physicians on an interprofessional team.[163] The notion of "integration" in integrative care adds layers of complexity, in that different providers will use different language as well as varying philosophical frameworks; for example, what a medical doctor might call, "kidney disease," a practitioner of acupuncture and traditional Oriental medicine might see as "wind imbalance." Strategies are necessary to help harmonize different practices, to create sufficient cohesion that there is a sense of a team approach, yet respecting differences so that there is truly integration between biomedical and CAM approaches. Strategies disclosed by interviewees seem to include administrative and political concerns, legal and liability issues, and attention to the different cultures the various professions may represent.

For example, one center director stated that the center pays all its practitioners to attend a weekly, 2-hour meeting. The agenda conveys the multiple tasks:

> Part is case-based, part is business-oriented, and part is process-oriented, working on our own stuff. That is a challenge, because there's a little bit of arrogance and self-righteousness that some MDs walk in with, and defensiveness in the others. The MDs have the top of the turf in the hospital, so that's the arena of greatest growth—how MDs and non-MDs interface in the medical setting where the MD has more sacred ground just because that's the way it is, and how we grow trust among ourselves so we can truly practice in an integrative way.

In addition to the weekly meeting, all fellows and faculty are involved in making clinical presentations in integrative medicine each month, and there are 2 weekend retreats per year.

A second center director, when asked how the center handled conflict, responded by saying that the center would "view it more as a difference in perspective in the care for patients that different providers have." The director analogized intraprofessional collaboration to physician referrals to specialists and then added: "The field is young; we don't have this hammered out—it's just a stage of integration."

A third center director noted:

> We're not modality oriented; because most of this work is not modality oriented, it's about change. We're about sustainable change on the healing pathway and core issues. In so doing we get the traditional Oriental medicine perspective, body-workers, a lot of health creation planning and deep work around whatever our patients' health objectives are and working with them toward that. . . . [As regards] team meetings, [we have] less conflicts in that arena (e.g., diagnostic interpretation, philosophy). In order to do deep work with patients, you have to do it with yourself, to appreciate it. You can't treat a depressed patient if you're more depressed than the patient.

Thus, self-care and attention to process by providers in the center reportedly helped reduce overt conflict.

CASE STUDIES: MANAGING LIABILITY EXPOSURE

During our interviews, it became apparent that many hospital attorneys were unfamiliar with liability issues pertaining specifically to inclusion of CAM therapies. Responses to attempts to establish integrative care ranged greatly, from mild concern to extreme caution. Most centers adopted a number of policies and procedures to help minimize liability concerns.

Case 6A: Reliance on Existing Hospital Strategies

Depending on the extent to which the integrative health care centers are integrated into the larger hospital or health care organization, a host of institutional, administrative, and risk management procedures and policies are likely to apply. Accordingly, some of the centers reported incorporating the general existing hospital-based risk management strategies to help reduce potential liability exposure. For example, just as risk management departments in hospitals review malpractice claims histories for conventional providers, a similar process is applicable to CAM practitioners. As one center reported:

> [I]nformation [concerning claims history] is maintained in a database and information is put in by our third-party claims administrator. Those names pop up when we run a credentialing report for our credentialing committee: whether it is litigation, or just a claim, etc. We work also with MSO [the medical staff office] regarding credentialing; they do more—run reports off the NPDB [National Practitioner Data Bank] for new applications for appointment to the medical staff, and for those seeking privileges.

The risk manager in this center reported that allied health practitioners are "rarely named in lawsuits," and CAM practitioners even more rarely: "Once in a while there's a suit against a midwife, but I haven't seen claims against chiropractors, acupuncturists, massage therapists."

In another center, the clinical director reported that risk management strategies are "no different in the clinic than the medical office," and include detailed attention to documentation in the patient's record. As to the potential for sharing liability risks with other members of the team, the director's response indicated a lack of concern: "If we comanage a patient . . . we'll have a conference about the patient. I've chosen to go into business with this guy, we're in business together."[164] In short, legal risks are accounted for but not overemphasized.

Case 6B: Coordination With Primary Care Services

Reliance on existing, hospital-based strategies is especially likely when the center uses one or more medical doctors, and particularly when offering primary care. Centers, however, differ on the extent to which they offer primary care, utilize medical doctors from the affiliated hospital, or depend on the patient seeing a primary care doctor outside the center. The decision to offer or not offer primary care may change the way the center views patient flow and the necessity for referral from or to a primary care doctor. Thus, the medical director for one center indicated:

> We have a primary care based practice here, so we follow primary care risk management practices, including a hospital manual, which is modified because we're off-site.[165] The hospital lawyers work with us mostly around contract issues, scope of practice, and risk management issues, but always using or adapting the usual hospital documentation—for example, how to properly discharge patients; how to comply with JCAHO requirements. . . .[166]

The medical director further commented on legal counsel's role in quality assurance and risk management as follows:

> We're up and running now and don't get checkups from counsel, though we're always subject to internal audit. We are compliant with JCAHO [the Joint Commission on Accreditation of Hospital Organizations]—our medical charting, the policies we set up, infectious disease control (sterilization techniques), confidentiality records—HHS [the U.S. Department of Health and Human Services] general practice guidelines, and NCQA [the National Commission for Quality Assurance]. We have a strict practice manager and the director of finance administration is strict too, to make sure we don't get dinged for anything. We know we're under a microscope—the center for alternatives; we have to be more clean than any other department or division. We took policies and procedures from the medical center side and added whatever we needed for us, worked with a business consultant who gave us other ideas, and created our own manual.

As a strategy parallel to relying on existing risk management strategies within the hospital, using hospital legal counsel, where necessary, and deciding whether or when the patient must visit a primary doctor, centers try to ensure that no conventional diagnosis or treatment has been overlooked.[167] In this vein, one center reported: "Each patient has an identified primary care doctor and their medical record, so that we are sure that the conventional bases are covered." Similarly, another center director reported: "I never envisioned [our center offering] acute care, so I honor conventional medicine, especially acute care."

Another center director explained the procedure for ensuring that patients receive appropriate conventional care: "We send patients to an MD who need to see them. But most providers are able to screen for problems requiring an MD." This director explained that every patient receives a consent form, which states: "I understand the treatment I receive in the complementary medicine clinic is adjunctive and does not replace conventional care." Following this statement, the patient must check off one of the following boxes: "I am under the care of a physician," or, "I am not under the care but am strongly advised to do so." The center worked out this language with the affiliated hospital's legal counsel, with the further proviso that patients who check off the latter box must be screened by a registered nurse prior to being allowed to receive treatment from a CAM practitioner. The director then clarified: "But 98% of our patients are under the care of a physician, so very few need to be screened."

A related risk management strategy involves soft-pedaling the availability of, and potential therapeutic benefit from, CAM therapies—

particularly as regards the inpatient setting. As one center director noted: "We don't do primary care in the clinic. We don't make claims about supplements." As regards internal marketing of services, he added:

> In the inpatient setting—transplant, cardiac surgery—we don't push CAM. We have a pilot study for guided imagery and music, using cardiac patients and their families. We don't push acupuncture or herbs; we used chaplaincy, bedside massage, and expressive arts—so we complement acute care. In the outpatient clinic, we're more change- than modality-oriented.

The center director further explained this risk management tool as an outgrowth of the center's core philosophy:

> Mind-body-spirit [definitions] are reductionistic in a way that trivializes the work, and nobody understands what they mean. I don't use the word *spiritual* often. I talk about inner, getting past the symptoms to the substance of the illness. We use those kinds of images and approach.

Within this philosophy, the center director reports having managed to respect the preferences of individual patient populations by making certain CAM therapies available. The director commented:

> A third of our patients are Asian, so on a doctor's order and a release, they can get acupuncture in the hospital, but most are content to wait until they get out. So we don't have acupuncturists and chiropractors wandering the ward. We have a study on acupuncture and stroke, and those patients get it—it's popular, everyone wants it.

Case 6C: Supervision and Quality Assurance

Some states mandate supervision of CAM practitioners under certain circumstances; for example, in some states, acupuncturists must be supervised by medical doctors.[168] Centers reported imposing supervision requirements with varying degrees of rigor (or lack thereof), but in general, interviewees did not share much concern regarding supervision of CAM practitioners within the centers, and there was little indication that legal counsel for affiliated hospitals emphasized a need for rigorous supervision. For example, one center administrator reported:

> When we brought in the non-MD licensed acupuncturist, he works under an anesthesiologist who works in the clinic; he is from China and knows more about Chinese medicine than her.

> There's informal dialogue but little actual oversight. . . . [The provider] has sent patients to him in the past and trusts him. The psychologist gets little MD supervision, because our medical director isn't here much.

Another center director reported that the concept of supervision is informal and that there are other quality assurance checks to help manage liability risk:

> Ultimately I'm supervising all the providers, as medical director, but we don't sign off on everyone's patient's visits. I don't see every patient; I don't sign their notes. Officially, a nurse practitioner has to work under a physician, although we never hammered it out. Everyone gets proctored (observe their exam, decision making, write-up), including physicians. This is a medical centerwide policy. . . . Then you get approved for full status and that's it. There's also quality assurance—I randomly review 5 charts a year and talk to the selected practitioners about their work. [As well, w]e meet once a week and go over cases. That's also a way to quality check as well as to learn a lot.

Thus, while supervision matters, it does not appear to be a major area of emphasis in management of malpractice liability risk. Rather, team processes and regular dialogue between providers serves to ensure that center directors are aware of how CAM practitioners are working with patients.

Case 6D: Institutional Scope of Practice

While scope of practice boundaries for CAM practitioners may be negotiated as part of the process of creating credentialing rules, they also are used as a risk management tool. Specifically, while the language of state licensing laws prescribes a specific scope of practice for each kind of CAM practitioner, institutions may choose, as a part of risk management, to further narrow providers' scope of practice.

In addition to narrowing institutional scope of practice, centers also may choose simply to defer including certain providers, out of concern for political correctness, or to allocate some modalities that are shared across professions to some providers according to what would be most politically feasible within the institution. For example, one center's medical director acknowledged using all of these strategies in combination:

> We haven't tried chiropractors—for political reasons; we're going for the low-hanging fruit first, until people feel comfortable with us.

Homeopaths—people will shoot water pellets at us if we bring them in, so we stay away from that, unfortunately, because I feel there's a lot of literature support for that. Energy healing—we tucked it under massage therapy and bodywork, they do it under the guise of that. Although we're explicit about the massage therapist doing Reiki in the case conference. Reiki is listed in the massage therapy list of protocols. Nobody has raised an issue about it yet. For now, the nutritionist doesn't do Reiki here.

In other words, controversial modalities such as energy healing are openly discussed in the inner circle of the team meeting (case conference), but not raised openly or defined for the hospital.[169]

A risk management director at the same center reported on the process in the following way:

A small group of us spent a lot of time coming up with standardized protocols for each of the practitioners—yoga, massage therapist (MT), chiropractor, acupuncturist—and they are detailed and lay out what they can and can't do. Cannot prescribe medication; make diagnoses. We set out the scope of their job duties and responsibilities and within their practice what they could and could not do. Those were approved by our initial Committee on Interdisciplinary Practice for the hospital. Those will go up the chain of command for approval by the executive medical board. . . . This was so new—developing and tailoring the protocols to different types of alternative therapies. It took some work but was not overburdening or overchallenging—it was everyone agreeing on the scope of practice and exactly on wording in each of those protocols.

A related question is how committees composed of medical doctors can justify agreeing to the scope of practice authorized by CAM practitioners' licensing statutes when the modalities such providers might use lack the same kind of evidence base to which physicians are accustomed. One medical director explained that her center uses a more expanded view of evidence-based practices than biomedicine typically acknowledges:

Our practices are evidence based. We recognize, however, evidence in the training of acupuncturists in information and knowledge they use in their occupational training. That is empirical cultural evidence that is recognized by the institutions. They are nationally boarded, so recognize their knowledge of herbs just as we recognize the gynecologist has to know of the medications that they will use in their practice. We do reviews of our training certifications and the medicines they use.

Case 6E: Continue to Monitor Conventionally

Recognizing that conventional monitoring is one way to limit potential malpractice liability exposure, one center gave examples of how its clinical model reduces legal risk.

> For example, asthma: We do a conventional approach and then talk about nutrition, adding these variables, such as stress reduction and breathing techniques. Our visits are eclectic, including suggesting acupressure points, doing manual diagnosis of myofacial dysfunction (we may refer to osteopathic physical therapists), and integrate whatever would make sense for a particular individual.

The medical director noted that in adding CAM therapies to the therapeutic armamentarium of its clinical staff:

> We use medication when necessary and often treat severe illnesses in a biomedical way while building the [use of CAM] so patients can use less medication over time.

Another center's medical director generally echoed the emphasis on conventional monitoring: "We do a lot of follow-up to ensure patients are safe. We have not had an adverse outcome, and are cautious about the treatments we recommend."

Case 6F: Awareness of Legal and Political Developments

While the integrative centers focus on patient care, medical education, and clinical research, they are not unaware of broader legal and political developments. For example, the medical director of one center noted:

> We've had five bills in the state legislature associated with CAM therapies. One is a health freedom bill; another is a due process for physician bill (having to do with adding integrative medicine to the state medical board). This is due to the state medical board harassing physicians who practiced CAM therapies in the last year. Another bill tried to make practicing CAM therapies a felony. Another bill, in response to that, tried to protect the folk healers in the mountains, but the sponsor is unfamiliar with CAM therapies the way we in the academic medical center think about it. The state already has a health freedom bill, but the board was not following the spirit of the law; apparently the board was moving mechanistically/in a mindless way and admitted it did not realize it has been biased, and that it did not understand integrative medicine. . . . There's a lot of paranoia on both sides.

Many doctors using CAM therapies are suspicious of the Federation of State Medical Board guidelines. The guidelines woke up the sleeping giants in our state medical board. For example, a physician doing chelation therapy got a complaint from a patient who claimed he charged too much—the complaint was based on the fee, not the care; the patient complained to the board; the board then subpoenaed his records, as well as associated laboratories. They asked the hair analysis lab to turn over records of what clinicians use their services; the lab refused; then a society formed to help fight the medical board.

Case 6G: Address Medical Errors

The director of risk management at a large institution pointed to use of risk management strategies generally as a first cut at minimizing liability in integrative care. These included the usual

> things to reduce possible claims and lawsuits, and [assessing] the amount we've paid [for various mistakes]: full disclosure to patients when a medical error has occurred; initiat[ing] conversations about compensation [when a medical error has occurred but] before the patient brings it up.

The director noted that there is a risk management staff member assigned to each department, and a person from each department who attends periodic morbidity and mortality conferences. As to integrative care specifically, there are "no additional restrictions or hurdles—we haven't had enough experience" (with claims).

Another center's medical director noted that the center will not offer "anything too invasive;" it will not "prescribe dietary supplements," but limits therapies offered to modalities such as Tai Chi, yoga, meditation, imagery, and massage. Whatever modality is recommended must be documented in the medical record, and any adverse event must be appropriately recorded. Further, in this center, patients need MD referral for acupuncture or massage therapy.

Case 6H: Test Outcomes and Modalities

One center's approach to liability management involved scrutinizing credentialing for specific modalities. The interviewee noted:

> On the hospital end, if there is a questionable treatment and a bad patient outcome and civil litigation, what is the hospital's responsibility? We could be liable on a theory of negligent credentialing: How

could you give the doctor privileges to do it? Or, another theory would be negligent oversight.

The interviewee gave an example of how the hospital handled a therapy lacking significant evidence, yet having strong political backing:

> We probably would not allow something like chelation therapy where there is no evidentiary basis to sanction it; we would not allow privileges for this modality. We retrenched at the medical board level because there was a lot of anecdotal testimony, including state senators; it's easier to not support it at the hospital level. We said if it's done at all it should be done in an outpatient setting elsewhere.

The interviewee clarified that there were two levels of analysis:

> One: What's an appropriate inpatient service? JCAHO says physician privileges should be site-specific. We need to know what we are physically prepared to invest time, resources, space, for. Maybe it's not cost-effective. Should the hospital allow any physician to do it?
>
> Two: Is this a procedure the particular MD has the requisite experience and training to do? We go through the departmental chairman: Is it a legitimate medical treatment, is it evidence-based, does the particular physician have the training and qualifications to do it? [We need to] maintain current competence and [ensure] that treatments are safe and efficacious. The chair makes a recommendation to a credentials panel (senior faculty) who review the physician's file; that goes then to the medical executive committee, and ultimately the board of trustees.

In short, a strong, well-developed credentialing process could be useful in managing potential liabilities for therapies with inconclusive evidence.

An attorney in a different hospital had a different perspective, commenting that the institution does not generally "review competency for many of the independent CAM practitioners, such as healing touch." The reason given was that "the questions are sporadic and it [the program] runs smoothly."

Again in contrast to this perspective, the administrator for a large hospital system commented that, in getting the CAM program operational, attorney support was critical: "We have 14 lawyers and they keep us in line." Before the program had full-time employees, its CAM practitioners were independent contractors, paid on an hourly basis, which raised concern within the institution. The hospital attorneys ensured that providers would receive an orientation "to make sure, for example, if you were doing massage therapy in a salon, that you knew these were patients with a medical condition, with platelet problems, with bleeding problems, that require ongoing medical sign-off." In this way, lawyers "have been involved every step of the way," from credentialing to liability management to reimbursement issues to "meetings with faculty and academic affairs people and finance people."

Case 6I: "Our Biggest Challenge Is Bureaucracy"

As a liability management tool, one center focused on the use of weekly case conferences to learn what conditions would benefit from various therapies. More specific strategies included the following:

> Patients have to sign a lot of forms: Most are [related to] HIPAA [the Health Insurance Portability and Accountability Act], consent to treatment (hospital), a history form, a two-page addition for us that describes spirituality issues and their own interests, goals.

When asked about the interaction with the hospital's legal counsel, and whether this positively or negatively shaped the amount of paperwork the center had to create to help manage liability issues, the interviewee explained:

> We created our own consent form and the legal department said it was fine. We go above and beyond by having our own consent form for each modality. Our counsel said we don't have to do this but it wouldn't hurt. There are a few modalities for which you need disclosure by state law and we incorporated some of this language. For example, with acupuncture we talk about minor bleeding and make sure the practitioner has had a conversation about risks and benefits. Each modality has a separate paragraph. . . . Other than that, the lawyers had no specific concerns. We would approach them and they were supportive and helpful.

Despite the positive report about interactions with lawyers, the interviewee noted that in general, there are layers of encumbering requirements within the hospital system:

> Our biggest challenge is the bureaucracy. We've been fortunate in maneuvering the political ladders. We learned if you ask for permission, it's easier if you just do it and ask later for forgiveness. Trying to do something as simple as offering gift certificates is cumbersome and difficult; getting different paint and carpet has been ridiculously cumbersome; posting for new positions takes a long time. Without a good administrator, we'd never have gotten off the ground.

Case 6J: Use A Screening Tool

One CAM practitioner, a massage therapist, noted that in addition to seeing patients in a separate room for massage therapy, the provider will "take a massage chair" and "help in surgical and overflow waiting areas." Risk is managed by using a "screening tool to make sure we're within the legal guidelines set up by the hospital." For example, if the massage therapy recipient is a nonpatient (e.g., a family member of a patient), then the institution needs to find out the person's identity and relationship to a patient; whether this individual has experienced massage therapy before; the recipient's level of stress; what kind of pressure they like in the massage session; whether they have any current medical problems; and what medications they are taking. The massage therapist does the intake and logs all the information at the center in case the recipients need treatment.

Another massage therapist at the same center mentioned the screening tool, and the existence of a weekly staff meeting to go over any issues and to provide supervision to the CAM practitioners. The center also is developing tools to share cases more formally between therapists.

In addition to the screening tool, scope of practice is limited in that the center asks its massage therapists to focus on inducing relaxation; deep tissue work is prohibited, though the massage therapist can refer to physical therapy. Healing work (or energy therapy) is, however, permitted, including Therapeutic Touch, Healing Touch, Reiki, and Sat Nam Rasayan, for which appropriately trained massage therapists and nurses can get credentialed.

The screening tool, like the consent form mentioned earlier, are standard ways that legal counsel in hospitals try to limit risk in conventional care as well. Our interviews probed whether center staff felt the requirements imposed on them were any more rigorous than in conventional care. Our sense was that there were not necessarily higher or different standards. For example, one center leader offered that every patient who receives acupuncture must sign a standard consent form. Under the relevant state law, the patient must obtain physician authorization for acupuncture; either the medical director authorizes the treatment or has the patient's primary care physician or nurse sign off that patient is receiving acupuncture. The interviewee felt this requirement helped the center administer care responsibly—"for example, it ensures that we're not trying to handle a treatable cancer with an energetic treatment." The center has a standard consent for treatment, plus specific consent forms for specific modalities and an informal (verbal) consent process for the CAM therapies (e.g., acupuncture, massage therapy, chiropractic).

Case 6K: "Everything Is Documented"

Another common theme in risk management was reliance on documentation and charting and the notion that the center must "handle risk management like any other clinical predicament." This center's medical director gave the example that "if a patient insists on using herbs, we document that the patient was advised not to do so and the patient refused." Within this center, the legal department "feels it's a continuum of care here so we don't need anything additional," other than a state law requiring that patients must sign a waiver when they receive acupuncture and must inform their physician. Legal counsel apparently found "little in the literature" concerning liability in integrative care.

This same center reported that regarding quality assurance, there were as yet "no adverse effects, patient falls, medication errors," or problems with therapies such as acupuncture. The director explained:

> We monitor clinical status and our providers are trained. We also don't look at moving nonexisting chi around and our therapies are explained from a scientific perspective. You want to walk the walk and talk the talk of the hospital. The hospital runs at a very high scientific level and we function accordingly.

By following the hospital's emphasis on the science behind various therapies, risk management matched the director's philosophical orientation. The notion of "working as a team" was also important for quality assurance.

Another center leader indicated that, at least annually, the center's practitioners are required to meet with the institution's quality assurance advisor to determine if any issues have arisen regarding safety, or if the providers are taking any new programmatic directions. For example, use of energy healing is "riddled with credentialing and ethical issues;" to assess its potential use, the center began by figuring out "what is it; what are the questions you should ask a practitioner; what does the literature say about it;" and where does the therapy fit in the Weiger grid— an analytical framework suggesting four quadrants of varying levels of safety or efficacy.[170]

Documentation also receives emphasis. For the numerous group classes and programs:

> we keep a "shadow chart" in our center on every participant and have a database so that at any point we can tell if our participant has completed our release, our screening tools, and in what programs (group activities) they have participated. If they do yoga, or massage, or acupuncture, we have them sign releases, more formal

and extensive documentation. Since we're open to family members we keep the "shadow chart" rather than a medical record for them.

As to inpatient acupuncture and body massage services, this center requires MD referral, and limits inpatient massage to "very light touch."

A CAM practitioner within this center commented regarding the inpatient service:

> We look at the patient record, platelet counts, what they are receiving in other treatments that may make massage contraindicated. In palliative care, for example, we'll get a list of people that are candidates for massage and we will visit with them and their families. Normally we do foot and hand reflexology, whatever areas we can work on—the healing touch, the warmth. They get chilled or crampy, and we try to help; also to be there for them in another way.

From this provider's perspective, the need to manage risk is balanced against the need to be present for patients as a healer, making sure the conventional bases are covered, yet offering "healing," "warmth," and the ability to "be there for them" in ways beyond the formal, medical care.

Case 6L: Use Independent Contractors

One center responded to risk management by making the yoga instructors and other therapists vendors or independent contractors and not employees. This approach is being taken by other centers that derive their income from vendor practitioners by leasing hospital space to them for their practices. The contract terms differ depending on who the vendor is (such as the instructor personally, or the instructor's institute). The hospital's attorneys are involved to ensure "these institutes for yoga are not putting terms in the contract with which the state will take issue." For example, the attorneys were concerned that "if someone claimed they were entitled to receive royalties for use of a particular healing method . . . we wouldn't want to have to suddenly pay for something where our patients wouldn't benefit." In this regard, risk management and credentialing concerns again dovetailed. The hospital attorney commented:

> We have contracts or memoranda of understanding with the independent CAM practitioners that are fairly sparse in terms of standard contractual terms. They provide, for example, their own liability insurance (if available). We assume many of these are low-risk activities. Our administrator is very cautious and has a number

of screening tools and only lets people in who are top-notch and embodies our values in terms of treating patients properly.

Another center also emphasized the retention of CAM practitioners as independent contractors, because "as a management team we want to limit our risk of employing them." In this center, the acupuncturist and chiropractor were the busiest, though neither had sufficient volume to be sustained full-time at the center. Financially, keeping these providers as independent contractors also helped pay overhead for the clinic, particularly as these providers increased their patient volume, enriching the center accordingly.

Case 6M: Manage Patient Relationships to Help Avoid Litigation

One lengthy interview was conducted with a hospital's attorney, who opined that there were few liability concerns and adverse incidents connected with the integrative health care center. Overall, "the administrator and her team don't seem to have any problems, so our intervention is minimal." In addition, the legal department "has a lot of demands for resources and the integrative health care center is not a priority since it does so well." Among other things, the center offers many lectures, workshops, and classes, which support patient education and self-empowerment. The attorney added:

> Liability risks are more a function of how patients feel about their relationships with their doctors and their hospitals, as opposed to the specifics of the care. The patient can get the best care in the world, but if the doctors or nurses are rude, the food is terrible, they can't find a parking space, they might file a claim over nothing; whereas someone who gets less than adequate care but feels their caregivers are trying may not sue.

The unhealthy dynamic of adversity between patients and clinicians seemed to be reversed in the integrative health care center:

> The patients are so fond and appreciative of our integrative health care center that it in fact adds to their good feelings about the overall institution and makes lawsuits less likely. The center focuses on the whole patient rather than just the disease; that contributes to a low rate of litigation here. We also have a patient advocacy department that resolves low- to mid-level complaints so they don't grow into litigation.

The attorney narrated one incident where a patient fell out of a massage chair and initially, "we had concern about whether they should have received a massage" at all. On investigating the incident, the attorney learned that the patient indeed had been "properly assessed and all appropriate fall precautions had been taken, so there was no negligence, just an accident that happened."

The attorney also put emphasis on avoiding therapies "that have a potential for physical harm (such as chelation therapy—injecting something into the body, See chapter 1)." In addition, practitioners are trained to "steer clear from claims about cure." Providers also are cautioned to "achieve a balance in terms of patient expectations," because, from the attorney's perspective, "liability comes from anger, which comes from being led to expect X and getting less than X."

On a physical level, light touch is recommended for inpatient massage to help protect patients who are frail, and who may have contraindications or risks. But—the attorney emphasized—the decision to limit massage therapy to light touch for inpatients came from the program itself, and not from legal counsel, another sign that the program is well-run. The attorney noted not only the strength of the integrative care program's administration, but also the positive institutional environment for the program's efforts.

By way of contrast, in another (rural) hospital, one provider mentioned the possibility of offering yoga and vitamins, and the docs looked cross-wise and said, "well there's no evidence." They had such hostility they could not envision what we do here. Here there are constant referrals, encouragement, support for yoga and massage, or at least patients get to talk about their interest in it freely. There is general acceptance of the role and value and the institution has supported this financially. That helps too from a liability standpoint—that docs aren't calling it voodoo.

MODEL STRATEGIES FOR MANAGING LIABILITY RISK

As suggested earlier, liability management and credentialing strategies often dovetail: A strong credentialing program reduces potential institutional liability, and knowledge of liability management should be part of what one looks for in hiring qualified practitioners.

Limits on PCP Status

One of the main questions is whether integrative health care centers are providing therapeutic approaches that are complementary (adjunctive) to conventional medical care, or are expected to take the place of the patient's regular medical doctor. This issue puts the centers in a bind, because many of the therapies they provide are not reimbursable, and many patients cannot afford to pay out-of-pocket. Unless the centers wish to cater only to the affluent, they must figure out how to coordinate care with the needs of many patients to receive regular, conventional care.

One of the risk management devices across centers—although rarely recognized explicitly as such—is the notion of the center as offering "consultative," rather than "primary" care. In other words, in its marketing materials and therapeutic approach, the center will explicitly disclaim any implied promise to provide the kind of front-line care a patient might expect from a primary care physician (PCP). Instead, the center will offer to consult with the patient's PCP, advising on complementary approaches as necessary.

Thus, in one center, a center leader noted that the medical director "serves in a consultative capacity" and "does not assume primary care of the patient and will refer [for this] to appropriate faculty." The medical director's role includes assessing patients for potential benefits from CAM approaches, overseeing the integrative care team, coordinating among medical and CAM practitioners, and ensuring that CAM therapies are "safe, effective and do not interfere with conventional care." This center offers a wide variety of CAM therapies including acupuncture, Chinese herbals, Tui Na (a bodywork technique within traditional Oriental medicine), biofeedback, counseling, massage therapy, nutritional and dietary counseling, and pharmaceutical and dietary supplement consultations. But the center does so in conjunction with the medical guidance from the patient's PCP. Similarly, in another center, the medical director noted:

> We are a consultative practice. Every patient must have a PCP to refer them. When patients try to self-refer, we have them get their physician to refer them. The PCP gets the treatment plan. We only see chronically ill patients who are frustrated with their allopathic care.

Some centers required that patients have on file, before their initial visit, a referral letter from their PCP; a softer version of this requirement is to have the patient leave contact information for the PCP on file. One center requests that patients have a referral from the PCP, "although many patients prefer that their PCP not be involved." Medical doctors within the center "do not act as PCP's, though." Some centers require referral from a medical doctor before allowing patients to receive acupuncture. In this sense, many such centers have imposed stricter requirements than state law; at present, few states require medical referral prior to acupuncture, or limit such requirements to patients being seen for serious conditions (such as cardiac conditions).[171] Many, to disclaim potential liability for missed primary care (and primary care diagnosis), required patient referral from a PCP; others offered to provide a PCP referral within the larger institution. Some institutions attempted to limit liability exposure by hiring CAM practitioners as independent contractors rather than employees.

But even in limiting provision of services to a "consultative" capacity, many centers still have unknown liabilities. To complicate matters, they are bringing together new kinds of multidisciplinary, clinical teams that have not been before in U.S. health care, for example, Reiki practitioners, neurologists, and acupuncturists or massage therapists, social workers, and herbalists. Cross-cultural communication between disciplines becomes increasingly important, as does the conveying of effective risk management strategies across the different professional groups.

Draw on Existing Hospital Policies

None of the centers reported any past or ongoing litigation involving negligent care by a CAM provider. Centers incorporated the general existing hospital-based risk management strategies (such as checking a provider's claims history) to help reduce potential liability exposure. These included:

- Developing use screening tools to limit potential liability from CAM therapies.
- Emphasizing conventional diagnosis and monitoring.
- Using multiple consent forms and waivers.
- Tracking connected legal and legislative developments in the state.
- Emphasizing evidence-based therapies and strong credentialing mechanisms.

Screening tools helped providers such as massage therapists in at least one center select which patients to disqualify from the CAM therapy, and thus help reduce potential liability risk. Screening tools for the CAM therapists thus served as a mirror to the provider's toolkit. Similarly, an emphasis on conventional diagnosis and monitoring helped counter the charge that inclusion of CAM therapies would put the patient in unnecessary danger; as noted, this is probably the most important of the liability management strategies.

Clinicians and administrators also seemed comfortable with rules governing documentation. Maintaining some consistency of documentation can be a challenge when including providers from different medical systems, such as physicians and acupuncturists. Few interviewees, however, mentioned difficulty translating records back and forth between clinicians, emphasizing instead the benefits of regular team meetings. Curiously, few referred to the Federation of State Medical Board Guidelines; these rules seemed to have had little or no effect on documentation requirements at the various centers. At least one interviewee mentioned related legal and legislative developments, though, and the need to parallel institutional efforts with such changes in the law. Finally, emphasis on strong credentialing mechanisms and evidence-based practice again served as a risk management device.

Decide on Necessity for Referral From or To Primary Care Doctor

Centers differed on the extent to which they claimed to offer primary care, utilize medical doctors from the affiliated hospital, or depended on the patient seeing a primary care doctor outside the center. In any event, centers attempted to ensure that the patient was receiving necessary, conventional medical care, whether within the center or elsewhere.

Avoid Claims About CAM Therapies

Centers helped manage potential liability by asking providers to avoid exaggerated promises of therapeutic benefit or minimizing claims regarding potential curative powers of CAM therapies. This posture also helps with compliance to Federal Trade Commission regulations.

Determine Necessity of MD Supervision

Centers differed on the extent to which MD supervision of CAM practitioners was necessary. In most, such supervision was an informal practice and not a required policy.

Decide on Whether to Narrow Institutional Scope of Practice

While scope of practice for CAM practitioners may be negotiated with key personnel within the institution as part of getting credentialing for CAM practitioners approved, placing institutional limitations on scope may be used as a liability risk management tool. Correspondingly, some centers may implicitly fold certain controversial practices (for example, energy healing) within the rubric of particular providers (for example, massage therapists), without articulating a formal policy to this effect; others may have expanded notions of evidence-based practice.

Use Team Meetings to Iron Out Conflict

Centers used case conferences not only to coordinate and exchange information concerning the approaches of different health care disciplines to patient care, but also to handle conflict between different providers, and thereby reduce the potential liability resulting from inadequate communication. Interviewees emphasized the benefits of clinical team meetings to iron out differences in care philosophy and to translate across diagnostic and therapeutic systems. Surprisingly, few (if any) described overt conflict in these innovative clinical teams. One explicitly noted that team members would work together to decide whether conventional care should bow, in a particular case, to a CAM therapeutic approach.

Manage Patient Relationships

Anger and adverse relationships often lead to liability claims against health care institutions. One attorney who was interviewed explicitly mentioned managing patient relations as a way to help prevent litigation. The interviewee, however, thought the center in question was well-managed and unlikely to generate significant liability exposure. Indeed, while clinician-interviewees generally expressed interest in the liability question, few seemed concerned with the possibility of imminent litigation. Presumably, having chosen to establish an integrative health care center, such interviewees either had already done their due diligence or had made the choice to work "within the system" to help reduce biases and establish new models of care.

Once again, though, models exist on an ad hoc basis, and the studies cited earlier with respect to credentialing[172] suggest that institutions are slow to build consensus models regarding policies to help minimize risk of malpractice liability exposure. For example, the 2005 descriptive study of 19 hospitals with integrative care centers found that there was no consistent pattern of liability insurance, either by provider type or between academic and nonacademic centers. This can probably be explained in part by the paucity of published judicial opinions concerning physician malpractice involving CAM therapies and the concomitant inability of legal departments in hospitals to make appropriate recommendations concerning precautionary levels of insurance. In any event, the ad hoc models discussed appear at least to create the institutional perception that liability risks can be contained and managed, thus permitting the spread of CAM therapeutic services within and across health care institutions.

CHAPTER 7

Empowering Patients

Effective Informed Consent

REASONS FOR INFORMED CONSENT

Many patients do not discuss their use of CAM therapies with their physicians.[173] This situation can leave physicians without sufficient information to assess safety issues, particularly regarding the possibility of interaction between CAM therapies and conventional treatments.[174]

The reasons for such nondisclosure are debated. According to one study, nondisclosure results from patient beliefs such as: "It wasn't important for the doctor to know" (61% of those surveyed); "The doctor never asked" (60%); "It was none of the doctor's business" (31%); and "The doctor would not understand" (20%).[175] Such lack of communication, whatever its origin, arguably impairs the therapeutic relationship and is compounded if physicians similarly fail to invite conversation. The situation also impairs patient autonomy interests in receiving sufficient information about therapeutic choices to make a knowing, voluntary, and intelligent decision about care options.[176] As Justice Cardozo noted, in articulating the doctrine of informed consent: "Every human being of adult years and sound mind has a right to determine what will be done with his [or her] own body."[177]

One potential consequences of poor informed consent is a lawsuit, as failed informed consent is another theory of malpractice liability. Yet little attention has been paid to date to informed consent governing CAM therapies. This situation leaves clinicians and institutions without guidance concerning the kind of written forms and verbal discussions that would help protect against unnecessary liability, yet respect patient decision making. Practices vary considerably.

SATISFYING THE LEGAL OBLIGATION

Few cases to date have applied informed consent rules to the arena of CAM therapies; yet in principle as regards informed consent, there is no particular reason to draw distinctions between CAM therapies and conventional care.[178] The standard for informed consent disclosure in conventional care is that the patient must receive whatever information is "material" to the patient's decision to undergo or forgo a particular treatment. The same standard theoretically should apply to CAM treatment: The clinician offering CAM therapies presumably is obligated to disclose to patients all the risks and benefits of such therapies that are material to treatment decisions.[179]

Under this rule, there are two standards for judging materiality in informed consent: About half the states measure materiality by what a reasonable provider would consider important to the decision to undergo or forgo a particular treatment, while about half measure materiality by what the patient finds important to making a decision.[180] Typically, in addition to a discussion of risks and benefits, information that is required to be disclosed includes such matters as the inability of the provider to predict results, the irreversibility of the procedure (if this is applicable), the likely result of no treatment, and available alternatives.

Failure to provide adequate informed consent is a second theory supporting malpractice liability (in addition to negligent care). To date, no patient has successfully argued that a provider's failure to disclose the possibility of using a CAM therapy, instead of a biomedical therapy, caused injury and constituted malpractice. At least one court has, however, observed that such an argument would succeed if the therapy in question had a sufficient level of professional acceptance.[181]

This appellate decision suggests that CAM therapies that are well-supported by evidence of safety and efficacy are potentially material treatment options and that therefore, the availability of such therapies should be disclosed to patients, as well as pertinent potential benefits and risks. Current clinical examples potentially include: use of acupuncture to reduce nausea following chemotherapy, which has been agreed to be effective by a National Institutes of Health Consensus Panel on Acupuncture; chiropractic care for acute low-back pain; and mind–body techniques for chronic pain and insomnia.[182]

Where patients are taking dietary supplements and also receiving conventional prescription medication, one could argue that informed consent implies a duty to inquire into the nature of those supplements, research any reported adverse herb–drug interactions, and advise or warn the patient accordingly. For example, adverse effects have been reported involving the combination of St John's wort and the medication Indinavir in AIDS patients;[183] the duty of informed consent, therefore, likely includes a requirement that the clinician inquire into the patient's use of supplements and disclose such adverse effects where relevant.

Simply signing a form does not necessarily mean that informed consent has taken place. Rather, the clinician must disclose the material risks and benefits of a treatment decision in a conversation with the patient and thereby meet legal requirements of informed consent; the form merely offers a way to document that this process has occurred.

CASE STUDIES: INFORMING PATIENTS ABOUT CLINICAL RISKS

Many of the institutions interviewed do not have formal policies concerning informed consent, although a number have informal policies and practices. Our list of case studies, therefore, is brief. While many handle informed consent through verbal conversations, an important risk management strategy in some centers involves the use of written consent forms for particularly risky therapies.

Case 7A: Standard Forms

One center director noted: "Every patient signs a standard permission slip in the clinic, for example, for acupuncture or another CAM modality." Another center director stated:

> The patient fills out the standard hospital-wide terms and conditions form (an informed consent), and also an informed consent form particular for here—this includes that (1) we're not a primary care practice; (2) they pay out of pocket; and (3) that these are alternative therapies and do not serve to substitute for conventional therapies.

Case 7B: "Legal Is Encouraging Me to Keep It Long"

Another center uses several consent forms: (a) a generalized, hospital clinic consent form; (b) an informed consent for treatment of complementary/integrative medicine (in which the patient, as described earlier, checks off whether receiving contemporaneous care from a physician); and (c) an informed consent form for any hands-on treatment (e.g., acupuncture, massage, biofeedback). The final form lays out risks, side effects, and benefits of the therapy. There is also a four-page intake form (demographics, medical history, psychological history, stress). This center's director noted: "I've wanted to condense it, to help patients who get irritated by the form, but Legal is encouraging me to keep it long."

MODEL STRATEGIES FOR HANDLING INFORMED CONSENT

Integrative health care centers use various model strategies for handling informed consent.

Use Informed Consent Forms Judiciously

Centers differed in their use of explicit informed consent forms and more informal conversations between providers and patients concerning potential therapeutic benefits and risks. In most, however, informed consent was highlighted as an important part of the therapeutic relationship.

Insist on Appropriate Documentation

Since clinicians cannot disclaim negligence, consent forms do not always protect them and their institutions from claims of liability. Further consent forms can be off-putting to patients. Since integrative care emphasizes the importance of the therapeutic relationship, bureaucratic forms to limit liability may be inadvisable. However, most clinicians we interviewed seemed to have felt comfortable with the forms given by their hospital administrator or legal counsel and the insistence on appropriate documentation of patient consent for every CAM therapy. Some centers have multiple forms, including consents for individual therapies. This approach seems consistent with the conservative guidelines of the Federation of State Medical Boards, encouraging extensive documentation regarding informed consent disclosure and discussion.

SHARED DECISION MAKING AND ETHICAL CONSIDERATIONS

Definitions of integrative health care offered in chapters 1 and 2 emphasized patient participation in shared decision making regarding choice of therapies. Shared decision making means that neither the clinician nor the patient alone has ultimate authority over therapeutic choices; rather, both share preferences and negotiate options that are mutually beneficial, consistent with the patient's autonomy interest and the clinician's obligation to do no harm.

Historically, many clinicians have regarded informed consent as a bureaucratic intrusion on the therapeutic relationship. Indeed, informed consent mandates disclosure of information to the patient. Shared decision making goes beyond mere disclosure—and particularly beyond the practice of having the patient sign a form agreeing to the chosen procedure. Instead, shared decision making emphasizes that shared conversation that follows the clinician's disclosure of various therapeutic options, including those CAM therapies that have sufficient evidence of safety and efficacy to be considered material to the choice of treatment pathway.

Informed consent is both a legal and ethical obligation, and shared decision making an ideal that more closely expresses what informed consent aims to do, namely, empower the patient in a way that is consistent with the clinician's ethical duties. As suggested, this ideal of shared decision making is implicit in the notion of integrative health care, and should be considered as an optimal endpoint beyond the model strategies presently being used by centers.

Ultimately, the clinician's task involves balancing the duty of nonmaleficence with patient autonomy interests in a negotiated exchange that respectfully incorporates patient perspectives.[184] A more thorough way of expressing this balance is by considering, in any given clinical scenario, the following seven factors:[185]

1. Severity and acuteness of illness
2. Curability with conventional treatment
3. Invasiveness, toxicities, and side effects of conventional treatment
4. Quality of evidence of safety and efficacy of the CAM treatment
5. Degree of understanding of the risks and benefits of conventional and CAM treatments
6. Knowing and voluntary acceptance of those risks by the patient
7. Persistence of patient's intention to utilize CAM treatment

Thus, for example, if the patient's cancer can be cured with conventional, although invasive, treatment (surgery) and the evidence for CAM is low but the patient nonetheless understands and accepts the risks and insists on trying CAM therapies, then the conclusion would be that it is ethical for the physician to allow the patient to try her regimen of CAM therapies so long as the clinician continues to monitor her condition conventionally. If the risk of the cancer increases past a tolerable threshold, the physician should intensify attempts to persuade the patient that it is time to return to conventional methods of treatment.[186] In any case, the clinician should be aware of pertinent evidence and be willing to consider any intervention (CAM or allopathic) that has an acceptable risk–benefit balance; the clinician's ethical obligation thus is to apprise the patient of acceptable options and make a recommendation that respects the patient's value system.[187] Such an approach aims to meet the legal and ethical obligation of informed consent while engaging the patient in shared decision making.

Notably, informed consent represents only one area in which legal rules and ethical values converge, and the foregoing ethical framework offers one way to harmonize interpretations of integrative medicine with classical ethical values, in that this framework presents a richer mix of criteria for evaluating the appropriateness of CAM therapies than the old dichotomy: Conventional equals ethical, CAM equals untested and hence by definition unethical. The Institute of Medicine (IOM) Report on Complementary and Alternative Medicine acknowledges the usefulness of the ethical framework reported previously and the validity of trying to find a stronger balance between the ethical values of nonmaleficence, beneficence, and autonomy than existed in a more paternalistic past.

The IOM report also highlighted two new values to take into consideration: medical pluralism and public accountability. With medical pluralism, the IOM report gave voice to the need for "acknowledgement of multiple valid modes of healing and a pluralistic foundation for health care," even if some CAM practices are "rooted, at least in part, in forms of evidence and logic other than used in biomedical sciences, often with long traditions and theoretical systems of interpretation divergent from those used in biomedicine."[188] Similarly, with public accountability, the IOM report observed that some CAM therapies "may have less kinship with technologically oriented, biomedical interventions and greater kinship with therapies at the borderland of psychological and spiritual care that are offered in professions such as pastoral counseling and hospice."[189]

The IOM Report went on to state:

> Without rejecting what has been of great value and services in the past, it is important that these ethical and legal norms be brought under critical scrutiny and evolve along with medicine's expanding knowledge base and the larger aims and meanings of medical practice. The integration of CAM therapies with conventional medicine requires that practitioners and researchers be open to diverse interpretations of health and healing, to finding innovative ways of obtaining the evidence, and to expanding the medical knowledge base.[190]

This request for openness is put slightly differently in another source:

> Many important questions remain to be sorted, such as the appropriateness of third-party reimbursement for CAM therapies, evaluation of quality of care (and, one might add, cost-effectiveness) in

the integrative model, development of appropriate institutional as well as regulatory policies, and the right synthesis of clinical, research, sociological, and legal perspectives that makes integrative care "clinically responsible, ethically appropriate, and legally defensible." But the process of finding balance may require still deeper relinquishment of old perspectives and a greater reconciliation of the various ethical imperatives that drive social and institutional policy. This process will help free the metaphor of integration from the seeming anchor of evidence to the more free-floating, less visibly authoritative, but nonetheless vibrant task of successfully harmonizing a current cacophony of perspectives on what the field is and what it may mean for our future health.[191]

In this way, and consistent with other recent investigations of ethics concerning use of CAM therapies,[192] the IOM Report and other sources are providing a new and broader launching pad than has previously existed for conversations about ethics in integrative medicine.

CHAPTER 8

The Supplements Question

Dealing with Dietary Supplements

REGULATORY ISSUES

The regulatory category of dietary supplements causes institutions (and clinicians) considerable confusion, both clinically and legally. A key to clarifying the legal issues is understanding the Dietary Supplements Health and Education Act of 1994, or DSHEA.[193] This statute, enacted because of overwhelming consumer interest in making vitamins, minerals, herbs, and other substances more freely available, changed the way the federal Food and Drug Administration (FDA) regulates these substances. Essentially, the DSHEA affirmed that dietary supplements are to be regulated essentially as foods, and not drugs. This means that as a general proposition, so long as they do not make impermissible claims linking their products to treatment or cure of disease, manufacturers of dietary supplements do not have to prove safety and efficacy prior to marketing and distributing dietary supplements interstate.

The legal definition of a dietary supplement is:

a product (other than tobacco) intended to supplement the diet that bears or contains one or more of the following ingredients: (A) a vitamin; (B) a mineral; (C) an herb or botanical; (D) amino acids; (E) a dietary substance for use by man to supplement the diet by increasing the total dietary intake; or (F) a concentrate, metabolite, constituent, extract, or any combination of any ingredient described in clause (A), (B), (C), (D), or (E).[194]

Three examples of popular substances meeting this definition are echinacea, gingko, and St John's wort (chapter 9). These dietary supplements can be found on the shelves of most pharmacies as well as health food stores.

Manufacturers do not need to register themselves nor their dietary supplement products with the FDA before producing or selling them. At present, no FDA regulations specific to dietary supplements establish minimum manufacturing standards, although the FDA has repeatedly stated its intention to issue regulations on good manufacturing practices (GMPs) in the future, to help ensure the identity, purity, quality, strength and composition of dietary supplements.[195]

Many people make the mistake of thinking that DSHEA leaves dietary supplements unregulated. This is not true, although it is true that because of DSHEA, the extensive, premarketing testing requirements required for new drugs do not apply to dietary supplements. However, under DSHEA, a dietary supplement is considered unlawfully adulterated, if it presents a "significant or unreasonable risk of illness or injury" when used as directed on the label, or under normal conditions of use. In addition, the secretary of health and human services has authority to remove from the market a dietary supplement that poses an imminent hazard to public health or safety. But, whereas with new drugs, the manufacturer has the burden of proving safety and efficacy in advance of marketing approval, with dietary supplements, the U.S. government has the burden of proving that the product is unsafe and must be taken off the shelves, after the fact.

One important aspect of regulation under DSHEA concerns the labeling of dietary supplements. Under federal law, labeling includes what goes on the packaging, inserts, and the promotional material distributed at the point of sale. With passage of DSHEA, there now are several kinds of claims a manufacturer can make in labeling a dietary supplement, the most common being a disease claim, a health claim, a structure-function claim, a general well-being claim, and a nutrient claim.

Briefly, a *disease claim* suggests that the dietary supplement is intended to diagnose, treat, mitigate, cure, or prevent a specific disease (for example, stating that a product, such as St John's wort, treats depression). A *health claim* characterizes the relationship between the product and a disease or health-related condition (for example, the relationship between calcium and osteoporosis). One important innovation that DSHEA established was the so-called *structure-function claim*. This kind of claim characterizes the documented mechanisms by which the product acts to maintain the structure or a function of the body (for example, "fiber maintains bowel regularity" or "calcium maintains strong bones"). The structure-function claim is quite common among dietary supplements and allows manufacturers to make a statement linking the dietary supplement to health, without violating the prohibition against making disease claims. Related to this claim is the *general well-being claim*, which describes the general well-being that a consumer might expect to experience from consuming the product. A *nutrient claim* describes a benefit related to a classical nutrient deficiency disease (for example, vitamin C and scurvy).

There are various legal requirements for each kind of claim. For example, a health claim must be preapproved by the FDA before it goes on the label and must be supported by "significant scientific agreement" among "qualified scientists," that the "claimed link" between the product and the disease is valid. A structure-function claim must have scientific substantiation that the statement is truthful and not misleading. Further, such a claim must be accompanied by a disclaimer, which alerts the consumer that the FDA has not evaluated the claim and that the product is not intended to "diagnose, treat, cure, or prevent any disease." Unlike the health claim, the structure-function claim need not be preapproved by the FDA. But again, if a dietary supplement does contain a disease claim on its label, the product is subject to regulation as a drug, which means the manufacturer must show safety and efficacy prior to interstate marketing and distribution.

In actual practice, it may be difficult for the consumer (or clinician, or health care institution trying to set policy) to distinguish among these different kinds of claims. It is hard to tell, for example, why a claim such as "for the relief of occasional sleeplessness" would be acceptable, but a claim with similar language, such as "helps you fall asleep if you have difficulty falling asleep" would be unacceptable. According to the FDA regulations, the latter is a disease claim, implying that the product treats a disease or condition, insomnia, while the former is a structure-function claim. The lines between the two, though, are difficult to distinguish.

Moreover, increasingly, companies are blurring the boundaries of these different kinds of claims, by manufacturing and marketing what they call *nutraceuticals*. This term is not regulatory but an industry term used to describe and sell these products. Nutraceuticals, which sounds like "pharmaceuticals," is meant to imply that the product both is nutritious and contains properties that support health. The category includes medical foods, dietary supplements, and what are now called *functional foods*—foods that incorporate dietary supplements. For example, companies might sell potato chips, pretzels, or soft drinks that contain St John's wort or gingko.

It probably would be difficult for anyone without specialized knowledge about botanicals to understand whether such so-called dietary supplements, when added to foods, have any clinically therapeutic effect. Nonetheless, present legal rules would allow marketing of such nutraceuticals without prior FDA approval of the claim on the label (so long as it falls within the acceptable parameters previously described).

All of these circumstances complicates attempts by health care institutions to respond to patient requests concerning dietary supplements and to help clinicians decide how to address such requests. With clarity around relevant rules, they can better inform patients about the meaning of statements on the labels of the dietary supplements. Informed clinicians also can better advise patients as to risks and what relevance the claims on the label may have, if any, to potential therapeutic benefits.

As a final note, the FDA, a federal agency, has no jurisdiction over the practice of medicine, which is a matter of state and not federal law. This distinction means that presumably the FDA has no jurisdiction over what is said between provider and patient concerning dietary supplements. Nonetheless, each state has its own version of the federal laws that the FDA enforces. Further, state regulatory agencies may intervene if practitioners make excessive claims regarding dietary supplements or subject their patients to harm by recommending such supplements. Some states regulate potential conflicts of interest by putting limits (or prohibitions) on practitioners' sales of dietary supplements; in addition, some federal as well as many state laws prohibit certain kinds of financial arrangements between providers and clinics in which they have a financial interest.[196] The American Medical Association Council on Judicial and Ethical Affairs has also placed voluntary restrictions on physicians providing dietary supplements in their offices.

All these rules require careful attention by legal counsel familiar with the provider's precise circumstances. Moreover, although as suggested, the essential regulatory treatment of dietary supplements under DSHEA appears fairly stable, the FDA is constantly innovating and refining its regulatory approach in an effort to meet its mandate to safeguard consumer safety. Thus, it is useful to review the FDA's Web site as a resource for continuing guidance whether one is dealing with dietary supplements or medical drugs and devices. Whether the FDA's regulatory efforts err too far in one direction or another—that is, in the direction of tightening regulation or in the opposite line of increasing consumer access—remains a subject of continuing debate.

RESPONDING TO PATIENT USE

Some professional organizations are now beginning to implement guidelines governing patient use of dietary supplements in conventional medical settings. For example, the American Society of Anesthesiologists issued a recommendation that surgical patients taking herbal medications stop taking these products at least 2 weeks prior to elective surgery if possible; (2) prior to surgery, patients consult their doctors regarding dietary supplements; (3) patients who have questions about potential herb–drug interactions should contact their primary care doctor.

Several comments bear noting. First, the society has assumed that primary care doctors have (or should have) knowledge concerning the dietary supplements patients might use and potentially relevant herb–drug interactions. Second, the society cautioned that: "use of herbal medications is not necessarily a contraindication for anesthesia." In other words, the recommendation did not necessarily disallow surgical patients from using dietary supplements. Third, the society also issued a disclaimer that its suggestions were meant to enhance patient safety, but could not guarantee a specific outcome. The society thus mixed a quasi-legal caveat in its clinical guidance. Clearly, clinicians and institutions would benefit from staying abreast of similar, current developments in relevant professional organizations.

INFORMED CONSENT, CONFLICTS, AND INSTITUTIONAL POLICY

Beyond the society's guidance, clinicians could follow the informed consent and shared decision-making suggestions offered earlier. For example, clinicians may wish to counsel their patients regarding: (1) known toxicities and adverse events associated with a particular dietary supplement the patient is currently taking; (2) any medical evidence relevant to safety and efficacy (or lack thereof), as well as the documented mechanism of action; (3) the fact that anecdotal reports concerning the dietary supplement's effectiveness do not constitute medical proof of efficacy.[197]

Clinicians (in addition to pharmacists) should be mindful of the distinctions made by federal regulations about the different kinds of labeling claims. Most nonphysicians, as noted, are not allowed to prescribe drugs. And although dietary supplements are in a different regulatory category under federal food and drug law, cases have been brought against nonphysician clinicians who have recommended dietary supplements, on the theory that these clinicians have prescribed "drugs."

Furthermore, it may be troubling that federal law treats a dietary supplement with a disease claim as a drug. Nonphysician clinicians who use dietary supplements to help treat disease could, in a worst-case scenario, be viewed as having crossed the line into practicing medicine unlawfully. It may therefore be wise for clinicians (and pharmacists) to limit claims about the therapeutic benefits of dietary supplements to what is stated on the label. This caution should not, of course, prevent (1) honest conversations about potential clinical risks and benefits and (2) disclosure and discussion about what may be unknown about the products (and their potential interaction with other therapeutic agents), as well as what is known.

Clinicians and institutions also should be aware of laws and regulations, if any, within their own states, governing recommendations concerning, and sales of, dietary supplements. For example, in addition to the legislative scope of practice limitations (discussed in chapter 5 for various CAM practitioners such as chiropractors) and related to giving patients dietary and nutritional advice, some states have rules governing clinicians' sales of dietary supplements.

Some of these rules apply equally to dietary supplements and pharmaceutical drugs. For instance, New Jersey provides: "A physician shall not dispense more than a 7-day supply of drugs or medicines to any patient. The drugs or medicines shall be dispensed at or below . . . cost . . . plus . . . 10%."[198] Clinicians who directly sell dietary supplements to their patients, and thereby earn a profit, may be perceived by juries as reckless and greedy, and find themselves liable for punitive damages as a result.[199]

Health care institutions also have to decide how to handle patient use of dietary supplements, particularly in the inpatient setting, even apart from use during surgery and scope of practice. As a starting point, institutions must decide whether to have a formal, written policy regarding dietary supplements or to simply have an informational resource (such as a library, a knowledgeable person within the hospital pharmacy, or a Web site) within the institution, or otherwise available, to respond to provider requests and, if appropriate, help initiate educational courses for clinicians.

The next step is to decide whether to include dietary supplements in the outpatient or inpatient formularies, and if so, what criteria to use to decide what products and brands to stock. Commonly used supplements, such as echinacea and St John's wort, might be more acceptable than unfamiliar herbs. Manufacturers of certain brands may have a better reputation for quality control and good manufacturing practices than others.

A related issue is whether to confiscate dietary supplements during patient admission, or establish criteria to determine which dietary supplement products patients might continue using, from their home supply, during hospitalization. These decisions are likely to require legal as well as clinical input and to involve multiple decision makers within the institution to fashion a policy that responds to patient interests while honoring clinical sensibilities.

CASE STUDIES: CRAFTING DIETARY SUPPLEMENT POLICIES

The task of setting institutional policy concerning dietary supplements seems to elude many centers. This deficit may exist because the contents of dietary supplements are not standardized, or clinicians and centers lack means of quality assurance comparable to that afforded pharmaceuticals. Furthermore, although the FDA, a federal agency, has no jurisdiction over the practice of medicine (which is governed by state law), the FDA occasionally has taken enforcement action against clinicians who have offered their patients dietary supplements that the FDA suspects are unsafe and ineffective. Potential adverse herb–herb and herb–drug interactions also are of increasing concern in the medical community.[200] For these reasons, there is probably the least consensus in centers regarding practice parameters around policies involving dietary supplements, with many centers leaving policy to the individual clinician.

The interviews concerning dietary supplement policies did reveal certain common ground but with considerable variation. Centers varied as to whether they had (or lacked) formal, written policies concerning dietary supplements. Interestingly, none of the centers interviewed to date mentioned concern about financial conflicts of interest involving sales of dietary supplements, a topic that has been of increasing note, particularly among physicians.[201]

Case 8A: "One-Stop Shopping"

One of the centers that has no formal, written policy on dietary supplements stated that the main reason for lacking such a policy was that the center had just hired its medical director and therefore was only beginning to have discussions concerning use of herbal medicine. Further, the center had quality concerns: "We want to make sure the patients acquire the stuff (sic) that we know are known, tolerated, [and contain] no heavy metals, adulterants, in the product." He noted that although Chinese herbs were readily available in the population, they lacked quality control:

> There are desiccated products from Taiwan, which is different than your herbalist picking roots from various drawers and making you material for a tea. Those may work.[202]

Assuming some progress could be made toward quality assurance, the pharmacy director indicated that the center leadership desired to offer "some one-stop shopping" for its patients, by including vitamins, minerals, and "phytomedicinal herbals (saw palmetto, typical ones)." Thus, politics and marketing, as much as scientific and medical concerns, are driving institutional policy development. As regards concerns about efficacy, the pharmacy director concluded that safety trumps efficacy, noting:

> Whether it [the dietary supplement] works or not is between the patient and the provider; I'm more concerned with safety than (with) efficacy. I won't get into the ecumenical discussion. If we want to provide it, we'll do so in a way that is safe for the patients.

In addressing the mix of philosophy, liability concerns, business issues, and medical/scientific quandaries, the concluding question and answer suggest the extent to which the sense of the unknown permeates institutional policy. Thus:

> Q: "Do you worry about potential (presently unknown) adverse interactions with the patient's drugs?"
>
> A: "That's like worrying whether the earth will get slammed by a huge meteorite. . . . There's nothing I can do if I don't [know] about it."

Case 8B: Information Available

The medical director for another one of the centers offering dietary supplements to its patients indicated that there was no registered pharmacist on-site with expertise regarding dietary supplements; the center, however, had an informal policy or practice as follows:

> We make information available to providers through a proprietary Web-based database called Natural Comprehensive. This database prints information for providers as well as for patients. It helps educate them in shaping evidence-based practice. It is written by a pharmacist for the medical community, and discusses efficacy, dosing, toxicity, etc. It is updated daily and assists in counseling patients regarding dietary supplements.

Case 8C: "Long Way to Go"

Another center indicated that it presently lacked a written policy or protocol for handling patient inquiries concerning dietary supplements. The administrator commented that the institution

> has a 'long way to go' to allow herbs. The medical director is not real fond of herbs.

The administrator personally felt that, especially with an acupuncturist on board, "it's nuts not to have herbs." Indeed, the acupuncturist reported that he (or she) sometimes may see the same patient in his or her own clinic and recommend herbs in that clinical setting. One of the reasons the center had declined (or was unable) to formulate a policy involved the inability to determine and prove potency and purity of herbs: "We don't provide those services, and don't refer anybody because we don't know what other providers' services are."

Case 8D: Allow the Attending Physician to Decide

Yet another center allowed the attending physician to make an independent decision regarding therapeutic recommendations about dietary supplements. In one case, the parents of an infant patient were Asian "and wanted herbs, and we allowed that as an exception" to the general practice of declining to make recommendations. The same center indicated:

> We have a little store but it has nothing that Costco wouldn't have—supplements, CoQ 10. We don't use these for pathologic diagnosis—for example, [we might recommend] licorice for basic care of the gastrointestinal system, [but] not for ulcerative colitis.

Case 8E: Educate, Warn

In another center, the administrator reported that the hospital tended to ignore clinical decisions and policy involving dietary supplements and that he had to educate personnel and even "forced the pharmacy to put a warning about certain herbs." Among other efforts, he had succeeded in helping to create mandatory classes for all PharmDs and pharmacology students about herbal medicine. These programs spread to the dental and nursing schools as well as the medical school. The acupuncturist stocked herbal medicine and saw this as falling within his or her scope of practice, although the pharmacy itself did not stock supplements. Yet another center director reported:

> We don't serve herbs in the in-hospital setting: Those get confiscated like all other meds the patient gets. In outpatient care, our emphasis is not on herbs and supplements—which are just like pharmaceuticals, an excuse to take a pill, not dealing with diet, exercise, lifestyle, those things that make change.

The director thus articulated the view that dietary supplements are not core CAM therapies, but on the contrary, potential distractions from the true task of healing. The center thus equated dietary supplements with drugs, rather than viewing the former as "natural," "holistic," or inherently part of a holistic vision of health care.

Case 8F: "Work on Evidence-Based Practice"

One center expressed approval for using "some supplements, because many have become mainstream." The medical director gave the caveat, however, that with respect to dietary supplements, "we try to work on evidence-based practice, this is what we teach strongly to the medical students." This evidence-based approach then gets communicated to patients; the clinicians try to

> divulge . . . whether this [recommendation for supplements] is based on RCTs [randomized control trials], anecdotal or case control, and I explain to patients and students what I use and why. But I also look at the safety profile. If it is anecdotal but has a good safety profile I allow it (e.g., peppermint capsule for cramps and IBS [irritable bowel syndrome], or problems with gastric emptying). There may not be a large RCT to support it.

The medical director cautioned that "a lot of the therapeutic effect [from dietary supplements and other therapies] may be placebo-based, meaning we amplify whatever we use with the therapeutic relationship." The focus, therefore, was on "empowering patients to use their own resources, belief systems," yet being "careful in what I [as a clinician] choose [to recommend]."

The approach is slightly different in another center that involves both conventional and CAM practitioners in decision making concerning dietary supplements. This center's medical director noted that the center recommends supplements (and where to obtain them), but only as part of a 4-page treatment plan that is developed collaboratively by the MD and CAM practitioners within the center.

Case 8G: "We Snuck in Chinese Herbals"

One center that has both a practitioner specializing in traditional Chinese medicine (TCM) and an outpatient pharmacist noted that the pharmacist monitors for herb–drug interactions. As for the TCM practitioner, the administrator noted, "we snuck in Chinese herbals and are dispensing those but we've been strategic." The TCM practitioner, in conjunction with the pharmacy department, created the hospital's herbal policy. Curiously, the center does not offer or recommend any Western herbalism supplements such as gingko or St John's wort.

The acupuncturist and TCM practitioner at this same center described the path to convincing the hospital to adopt the policy on herbal medicine:

> I went point by point about myths and misunderstandings about herbal medicine: I noted it is unsafe when prescribed by people who don't know what they're doing, and when dispensed by companies that are not competent. With professionals it is safe. When patients get herbals outside the hospital, that is when safety issues arise.

The TCM practitioner, having established TCM's expertise regarding herbal medicine, then added:

> We have to keep the pharmacy out of Chinese herbs, because they know nothing about them, about doing an examination or asking the right questions. The pharmacy wanted to sell supplements, which would have taken it out of our hands; they would not know about dosing, or if the patient started to get loose stools with a particular formula—what does that mean. I pointed out all the lack of expertise in Chinese herbs and that therefore it is not appropriate for them to be involved. . . . We are strict about getting the herbs only through one company, which we felt after extensive research was reliable.

Even though the acupuncturist would be in charge of recommending Chinese herbs, the pharmacist "may recommend supplements occasionally, and helps answer questions about medication or supplements, or about adverse herb–drug reactions."

A second selling point was financial: "We also made the point that it would help generate revenues—sending patients outside the hospital would be a loss of revenues. The practitioner also clarified why the center does not offer the kind of Western herbalism dietary supplements commonly available in health food stores:

> We drew a line between Western herbs and supplements and Chinese pharmacopoeia. We (the acupuncturists) do not deal with Western herbs and supplements; our legislatively authorized scope of practice focuses on Chinese herbal medicine.

Despite this line, a clinic affiliated with the hospital has supplements in its pharmacy, but apparently "sells few because pharmacy personnel lack expertise in that area." Nonetheless, "they might have paved the way for us, though, by introducing the idea of herbals."

Case 8H: "We Only Research Botanicals"

One familiar theme in many of our interviews was the decision by centers to refrain from offering any herbal therapy for treatment, but instead emphasizing research into botanicals. One center noted that its Web site manager is a pharmacist who also has botanicals expertise. Some centers have specific concerns about dietary supplements—for example, the concern that in oncology, patients not use any botanicals while getting treated with chemotherapy, surgery, or radiation. In such cases, one or more centers might have its pharmacist or nutritionist on staff recommend "a USDA level vitamin-mineral complex, but not a vitamin per se" or any commercial dietary supplement.

Case 8I: "None Are Recommended"

One center leader asserted that as regards dietary supplements, "none are recommended." The question then arose of what to do if patients themselves initiated requests for, or had questions about, dietary supplements. This institution's response was to refer such patients to a staff pharmacist, nutritionist, or dietitian affiliated with the integrative care program but employed by the hospital. Within this institution, all such personnel are required to pass an exam developed "specifically on herbs and supplements" and tailored to use by the specific patient population drawn to the center.

Another center's research director explained that practitioners make recommendations but do not sell dietary supplements. Each provider makes his or her own determination as to which supplements to recommend (e.g., herbal formulas, remedies, vitamins). Meanwhile, the center's staff as a whole is developing patient education materials and standards to guide practice.

Case 8J: "We Go Undercover All the Time"

One center leader emphasized the need to learn what patients are told about dietary supplements outside the institution and to bridge these perceptions with the medical evidence. Thus:

> We go undercover as patients all the time to health food stores to learn about what they are advising our patients to take. It can be up to hundreds of dollars a month that they are selling per patient.

This center does not recommend dietary supplements, but it advises patients in response to requests for information, in two ways. First, "when patient approaches us about any ingestible," the center guides the patient to its clinical dietitian and to its pharmacist. Second, it directs patients (through these providers) to an evidence database to offer the patient information about the medical (and institutional) perspective. In this center, even the acupuncturist does not dispense herbal products. The center also writes up informational packets and distributes these throughout the hospital, to help "increase communication" between clinicians and patients, and train physicians to ask their patients about use of dietary supplements. Tools include an intranet system, with a commercial product known as Natural Standard, which gives information institution-wide about dietary supplements.

Another center, which also is active in the use of dietary supplements, has "an acupuncturist who uses prepackaged herbal pills, and a Western herbalist that also practices Japanese-style herbology." This center also sells vitamins and nutritional supplements for use in functional medicine.

The approach is somewhat different in a third center that also actively responds to patient interest in dietary supplements:

> On an outpatient basis, we recommend nutritional supplements, botanicals, but not in the truest sense—we're not herbalists. An herbalist would cringe to use single agents (which we use). Our training does include preparation of poultices and wild-crafting, but generally we use commercial herbal products.

In this center, therapeutic recommendations regarding dietary supplements are limited to outpatients. For inpatients, the pharmacy and therapeutics and other hospital committees would not authorize recommendations of botanicals, and "though we could agree to patients' existing choices," there were arguments within these committees about quality assurance and questions as to brands patients should be allowed to continue using.

Case 8K: Looking for Red Flags

An interview with the senior pharmacist for the hospital housing one of the centers yielded rich information about a relatively sophisticated approach to patient use of dietary supplements. In this hospital, there are about 40 clinical pharmacy specialists, each serving the different disease treatment sites or services within the institution (such as thoracic head and neck; GI; bone marrow transplant; breast cancer). Within the hospital, only pharmacy staff are allowed to dispense supplements.

The senior pharmacist expressed the view that most patients are "well-read" concerning dietary supplements—particularly in the breast and prostate cancer services, where they use these products widely. The hospital routinely asks patients, both as a new visit and in a follow-up visit, about all their medications including dietary supplements. Physicians, nurses, and other clinicians (as well as pharmacy staff) are trained to "be aware that people are taking these and that we need to have open communication with patients around this."

Typically, nurses do the first screening. If patients are on "more than vitamins," the nurses call the pharmacy staff, who then

> write down everything they're taking plus all the medication they are taking (e.g., for diabetes, high blood pressure, heart conditions). The pharmacy staff will review all the literature and try to review all the ingredients, looking for four to five "red flags":
>
> - High-dose antioxidants. Whether the chemotherapy will potentially rely on production of free radicals for their mechanism and the antioxidants might interfere (this red flag is largely a red herring).
> - Products that have hormonal properties (or have the potential to increase hormone levels) with regard to breast cancer patients. We take a conservative stance even regarding soy. We prefer they take whole foods than a powder.
> - Effects on coagulation, particularly in patients on coumadin. Our patients are at increased risk of clotting and low platelets if on chemotherapy.
> - Anything that could affect the immune system, either positively or negatively. For example, we have bone marrow transplant or even multiple sclerosis patients who may be on immunosuppressants, and we would not want to stimulate the immune system for them. However, some patients may be immunosuppressed and might benefit from such supplements.
> - We look to drug-supplement interactions, such as St John's wort and a certain chemotherapy that has been shown to interact with St John's wort. We look for supplements known to cause liver dysfunction or other safety issues (e.g., chaparral, pennyroyal oil).

The clinician's job then is to "talk to the patient about all the information, the pros and cons (risk and benefits)." The first focus is usually on safety rather than efficacy, because the hospital's position is that, if the product is safe under pharmacy review yet has questionable efficacy, then "it's up to the patient to decide whether it is worth the money to have that potential benefit (even if the evidence is not there to support it)."[203] If the pharmacy staff deems the product unsafe, it will "try to discourage but it's still up to the patient, their decision." The institution must document the patient's decision in the chart—"whether by dictating, writing the note, or putting it in an e-mail which we print and include in the medical record."[204]

When asked to evaluate the foregoing policy, the senior pharmacist indicated that the "system works well but it's time-consuming, especially for the physicians." To help alleviate the burden, the pharmacy staff provides support, such as responding to calls and looking up relevant information, and evaluating and reviewing the ingredients. The system does not work well when the patient is using dietary supplements from China that have unknown ingredients. The hospital has some staff who can translate the Chinese. The policy again is to respect patient choices as much as possible:

> If someone got the substance but we do not know what it is, we tell the patient, "If it were me I wouldn't take something with an unknown substance. If you're going to ingest it, you should know what it's in it." We outline the issues and the fact that there are some people out there who want to take advantage of them and others who sincerely believe the product but have no information about it. We lay out the concerns and it's the patient's decision.

Not all physicians comply with this autonomy-rich policy; some "tell the patient, 'don't take any of that,' " whereas others refer the patients to the pharmacy staff for more information. As regards potential liability issues, the hospital is satisfied in "letting patients decide based on information we give them, and then documenting that decision in the medical record." Yet even with this liberal policy, the pharmacists still "get flack from patients who strongly believe in their supplements."

MODEL STRATEGIES FOR HANDLING DIETARY SUPPLEMENTS

Because dietary supplements occupy a unique regulatory niche—between foods and drugs—and lack the quality assurance and standardization of pharmaceuticals, they leave institutions in a quandary. Some have adopted a bury-head-in-the-sand approach. Others adopt formal (written) policy, while many rely on more informal practices. Responses ranged from not offering any recommendations regarding dietary supplements, to having hospital pharmacies stock selected supplements. Yet another approach involved sticking to research on (rather than clinical advice concerning) dietary supplements; and a variation on this practice involved insisting on an evidence-based approach.

But centers also had highly varied solutions as to who could recommend what, often leaving a patchwork of policies regarding supplements within a given center. For example, one center had no pharmacist, but did have a naturopath who could make herbal and nutritional recommendations. In this center, providers could give the patient "names of Web sites for suppliers, or send them to a community pharmacy"; patients also could receive recommendations regarding Chinese herbal medicine from the acupuncturist and information about herb–drug interactions from the physician. Again, given consumer demand for supplements, loyalty to their chosen products and brands, and the fact that federal law allows access irrespective of scientific perspectives, the choices made by centers seem like efforts to confront an impossible dilemma: acquiesce to patient choices on one hand, or impose an unnecessary paternalism in denying those choices on the other.

Other than adopting a formal (written) policy, integrative health care centers use various strategies to handle dietary supplement practices.

Limit Recommendations to Products With Known Quality Assurance

Because dietary supplements—particularly, as reported in the literature, certain Chinese herbals—may be adulterated or otherwise dangerous, quality assurance is crucial, leading institutions to focus on manufacturers whose products are known to be of high quality.

Offer Informational Resources for Providers

Particularly because even providers who avoid recommending dietary supplements may be asked to respond to patient requests concerning specific products, some centers implemented an informational resource for providers. The informational resource may be within the hospital pharmacy, and may contain warnings regarding specified dietary supplements. One center included educational efforts in the curricula of affiliated professional health care institutions.

Limit Use of Dietary Supplements to "Wellness" Care

Although a principled distinction between wellness care and disease treatment may be difficult to sustain, centers may find it helpful to reduce reliance on dietary supplements as part of the treatment regimen, and focus instead on their potential role in maintaining overall health.[205] This posture would be consistent with the clinic director cited in the foregoing case study who equates use of dietary supplements with use of drugs for the management of medical conditions. This posture also applies to the next strategy.

Emphasize Overall Health Strategy

At least one center expressed concern that patients were taking dietary supplements in ways analogous to the "magic pill" of pharmaceuticals— a temporizing solution that potentially distracts the patient from the overarching goal of restoring emotional and spiritual balance. This center emphasized refocusing the patient on an overall health strategy, in addition to symptom relief and disease cure.

Emphasize Evidence Base

Once again, centers seemed to rely on the position of limiting therapies to evidence-based recommendations. They also attempted to communicate the evidence base to patients during informed consent and shared decision making. This involved translational efforts back and forth, as patients communicate information and preferences, and clinicians describe how those choices resonated or not in the medical literature accumulated to date.

Limit Scope of Practice

A stronger position involved limiting the scope of practice of selected providers, or even of all providers, regarding dietary supplements. More than one center indicated that dietary supplements may not be recommended by any provider. Others limited recommendations to a given practitioner's expertise—for example, nutritionists, pharmacists, dieticians, and acupuncturists may be able to recommend different kinds of supplements (such as multivitamins versus Chinese herbals). Some centers indicated that they would research herbal products, but again, not allow therapeutic recommendations.

Check for Adverse Reactions and Other Red Flags

An even more robust strategy involved finding out, as part of the history taking, what supplements center patients already are taking, and then emphasizing shared decision making as described previously. One center had a full-fledged system to check for red flags regarding potential adverse interactions with conventional medication, and for safety issues. This system, devised by the hospital's senior pharmacist, then allowed the center to put safety first, and make policy decisions accordingly.

The breadth of responses to issues concerning dietary supplements reflects the continuing debate about their appropriateness as a healing or potentially curative modality within the notion of integrative care. Once again, though, recent studies reveal that institutions have not yet emerged with a strong consensus regarding dietary supplements. Yet, despite this lack of consensus, the emerging ad hoc approaches discussed in this chapter represent sensible methods of dealing with the contrast between the ambiguities in research and clinical practice surrounding dietary supplements and the widespread availability (and marketing) of these products among health care consumers.

See Appendix D.

CHAPTER 9

Integrative Medicine for Pharmacy

Dietary Supplements in Practice

FEDERAL POLICY AND STATUTES

As presented at the public testimony of the U.S. House of Representatives Committee on Government Reform at their hearings on "The Dietary Supplement Health and Education Act of 1994: Ten Years After" in March 2004, much of the practice of integrative medicine is based on the availability of practitioners providing services, as discussed elsewhere in this book, as well as the availability of products classified today as dietary supplements as discussed in chapter 8. In this regard, appropriate information about, and quality of, materia medica is critical. Many of these issues fall under the category of pharmacy practice in general, and hospital formularies specifically, as applied to the health care system.

Legislative and Regulatory Environment

Critics often underestimate the extent of regulatory authority the federal Food and Drug Administration (FDA) can exercise over dietary supplements. Even the FDA commissioner, according to the House Committee on Government Reform, July 2001, has at times misunderstood the full extent of FDA regulatory authority. Prior to 1994, the FDA regulated dietary supplements as foods in most circumstances. With the passage of the Dietary Supplement Health and Education Act (DSHEA) of 1994 (amended in 1998), dietary supplements and dietary ingredients were regulated as a category unto themselves—neither as foods nor, as some wished, drugs. Under DSHEA, the FDA has the power to regulate the accuracy of information about and the safety and quality of all dietary supplements.

The FDA is capable of ensuring the accuracy of information used to describe dietary supplements in the following ways:

- By obtaining injunctions against the sale of products making false claims
- By suing any company making claims that a product cures or treats disease

To ensure the safety and quality of dietary supplements, the FDA also has the power

- to require good manufacturing practices (GMPs), including ingredient identity and product potency, cleanliness, and stability (although it was not until 2003, some 9 years after passage of DSHEA, that the government published proposed GMP rules for dietary ingredients and supplements, and these rules are still not expected to be finalized until sometime in 2007);
- to refer the sale of toxic or unsanitary products for criminal action;
- to seize products posing an unreasonable risk of illness and injury;
- to stop sales of entire classes of products if they pose an imminent health hazard;
- to stop products from being marketed if the FDA does not receive sufficient safety data in advance under generally recognized as safe (GRAS) provisions.

Nonetheless, the health care system must rely on vigilance by the medical profession and voluntary compliance by industry in safeguarding patients against adverse reactions. Following the congressional elections of 2004, changes had not been anticipated in the Dietary Supplement Health and Education Act, which would continue to regulate herbs as dietary supplements, not as drugs. In his memoir, Sen. Orrin Hatch (R-Utah), cochair of the Congressional Caucus on Complementary and Alternative Medicine and Dietary Supplements documents the unprecedented involvement of a coalition of citizens and commercial groups in the passage of this bill.[206] However, there have been changes in the 2006 session of Congress in the organization and composition of the caucus with consultations among Sen. Hatch, Sen. Tom Harkin (D-Iowa), and Sen. Richard Durbin (D-Illinois) about future legislation on dietary supplements. Two initiatives articulated by Sen. Harkin have been to allow dietary supplements as an itemized medical deduction for income tax purposes and to allow purchase of dietary supplements with food stamps.

It is likely that what may not be achieved by more legislation and regulation may be helped by better information and education of consumers and health professionals. It is also necessary to work with an active and growing natural products and dietary supplements industry in the United States. Some responsible natural products suppliers, manufacturers, and distributors are beginning to recognize that the integration of herbal and nutritional medicine into medical practice mandates higher standards of product ingredients and information about their efficacy. The practice of herbal medicine has generally been conducted as part of ambulatory care[207] as consistent with the general limitation to outpatient services of the centers described in this book.

RESEARCH EXPERIENCES WITH SPECIFIC HERBAL REMEDIES

As integrative medicine moves into mainstream practice environments, there are opportunities to carry out studies on hospitalized patient populations. While this development may add to the evidence base for the use of dietary supplements,[208,209] in some cases ignorance of the historical usage of herbal remedies may lead to inappropriate studies.

St John's wort, gingko biloba, kava kava, and ephedra have all come under scrutiny in recent years and each illustrates a different aspect of the expanding use of herbal remedies as information, and in some cases, misinformation comes to light.[207,208] Such opportunities had not existed until herbal medicine became accepted as a subject for mainstream medical research. Faulty conclusions may result from studying the dietary supplement in an inappropriate population, or with an inappropriate dose or schedule (by ignoring historical use) regarding efficacy, or by inappropriate assessment of side effects regarding risk. Each of these circumstances has applied to recent, high-profile research on four popular and historically effective dietary supplements: St John's wort, ginkgo biloba, kava kava (or kava), and ephedra.

St John's wort (SJW) has long been considered under historical use an effective treatment for mild to moderate depression. One study tested SJW on patients with depression sufficiently severe to be hospitalized. There has been no practical experience on what the appropriate dosage or regimen might be in such patients. The study found SJW to be ineffective (the conventional antidepressant was also ineffective in this study) while depriving patients of needed psychotherapy when there was no plausible reason to believe that SJW might be appropriately used in this population.[210] Consequently, a question is raised about the ethicality of such an experiment in the first place. Another question was raised about adherence and compliance among the treatment and control groups as measured by hyperforin (active ingredient of SJW) as a marker.[211] Subsequent clinical studies on SJW[207,212,213,214] as well as meta-analysis and comparative studies[215] have shown generally positive effects in treatment of mild to moderate depression and uncovered methodological issues in previous studies, such as members of the placebo groups having SJW active ingredients in the bloodstream (secular trend), and members of the treatment group *not* having SJW in the blood (compliance) in additions to difficulties with dosage and dosage schedule.

It is important not to ignore "historic use" when moving herbal remedies into the mainstream. Another study widely reported during 2002 showed no difference between placebo and conventional medication in severely depressed patients who were also given 14–16 hours of intensive personal care from highly trained mental health professionals. Perhaps the real message for severe depression is that neither herbs nor drugs alone can effectively substitute for hands-on therapeutic care, which is consistent for some of the strategies adopted by the cases illustrated in chapter 8.

Gingko biloba is well established as an effective treatment for mild dementia and has been demonstrated to improve memory in those with documented memory impairment. However, it has been marketed irresponsibly as a generic memory enhancer, leading to a misguided study of gingko using standard tests of memory in those without cognitive impairment.[216] The subsequent promotion of the negative findings on gingko in this study have led to great confusion.[208,217] Again, historic use has been ignored to the potential peril of researchers, study participants, and the general public. Studies on the safety of gingko and drug interactions continue.[218]

Kava kava has had historic experience in approximately 70 million people for use as a muscle relaxant and sleep inducer.[208] In June, 2002, the BfArM (German Federal Institute for Drugs and Medical Devices) had issued an official letter immediately revoking the marketing authorization of kava. The letter declared this measure to be based on a revised benefit–risk ratio mainly resulting from 37 suspected cases of adverse effects of kava on liver function. The letter stated that a high risk of "severe, life threatening adverse effects on the liver" has to be expected with kava intake.[219] Liver toxicity is not uncommon with many prescription and over-the-counter (OTC) drugs; there are hundreds of deaths due to liver failure each year from the routine OTC use of acetaminophen, for example.[220] In a case-by-case analysis of the kava finding, however, investigators found several alternative explanations for the 37 suspected cases of liver toxicity in those taking kava, and concluded that those cases cited by the BfArM are highly questionable.[221]

As an effective treatment for anxiety and insomnia, should kava be banned or should there be developed a responsible approach to risk–benefit as with other treatments manifesting side effects? The case-by-case analysis by Gruenwald and colleagues[221] found alternative explanations for liver toxicity in those taking kava kava. Nonetheless, many retailers have voluntarily taken kava kava off the shelves in response to these claims, demonstrating the public loss of a potentially valuable dietary supplement based on research that is not scientifically sound.

Ephedra had been used by millions for weight loss and was also inappropriately used as an athletic performance enhancer.[208] Its being listed on autopsy reports as contributory to several fatalities among otherwise healthy individuals has led to its restriction. An FDA-commissioned report in 2003 stated in its final ruling that 5 deaths could be attributed directly to ephedra. To put this number in perspective, the American Herbal Products Association reports that approximately 12 to 17 million people took ephedra in 1999. The *Nutrition Business Journal* estimated that 2001 ephedra sales were $1.25 billion.[222] Regardless, these fatality reports led to ephedra being taken off the market in 2004, although the ban did not affect the sale of OTC decongestants, which often contain a synthetic constituent of ephedra, ephedrine. (There has subsequently been a movement to place synthetic ephedrine-containing remedies behind the pharmacy counter.)

It was not until 2005 that a Utah-based nutraceutical corporation successfully challenged the ephedra ban, leading to a ruling that, in accordance with DSHEA, the FDA could not place the burden to prove safety on dietary supplement manufacturers as it does for drug and device makers. The court allowed the sale of ephedra products containing less than 10 mg of ephedra.

At the same time, the federal government has also cited obesity as a major risk factor for many diseases, while effective weight loss regimens elude many overweight individuals. It remains unresolved whether it is possible to have safe, medically supervised application of appropriate ephedra formulations for weight loss, or whether ephedra has no place whatsoever in contemporary use.

ADULTERATION

The further abuses of herbal products adulterated with therapeutic drugs and contaminants (especially a problem with imports from overseas, particularly China) represent a serious safety issue. Consumers, health professionals, and responsible elements of the U.S. natural products industry all suffer when irresponsibly adulterated products are imported from abroad. The National Institutes of Health (NIH) clinical trial on the Chinese herbal formulation PC-SPES for prostate cancer was undermined by the unwitting use of adulterated herbs.[223] Some natural products from China have even been contaminated with dangerous antibiotics such as chloramphenicol,[224] which may lead to bone marrow aplasia. Improvements in manufacturing and marketing standards in the natural products industry will be required for effective integrative medical practice.

INTEGRATIVE MEDICAL PRACTICE

Reliance on the appropriate use of nutrients and herbs is a critical and fundamental component of some integrative medical practices. Presently in the United States, these natural products are widely available. Unlike pharmaceuticals, information about the health effects can *not* be provided on the product label or with the product as a product insert. Due the increasing availability of credible third-party research on the efficacy of herbal and nutritional ingredients, and increasing recognition by the medical profession of the importance of dietary supplementation for optimal health, and for the prevention and management of many medical conditions,[225,226] it is incumbent on practitioners of integrative medicine to maintain a medical standard of information and practice about herbal and nutritional ingredients. One approach to this requirement is to develop and maintain capability for a clinic- or hospital-based formulary of appropriate, effective, and high quality sources of herbs and nutrients.

The current regulatory environment is coupled with the reality that much of the natural products industry does not operate to medical and scientific standards, that many irresponsible marketing claims are made, and that many medical and scientific professionals are not knowledgeable about the science behind herbal and nutritional medicine.

This volatile mix produces much confusion and misinformation on both sides, documented periodically by such influential sources as the *New England Journal of Medicine*[217] Medical professionals have been largely on their own in trying to understand the proper indications, ingredients, and dosages for the appropriate scientific use of herbal and nutritional remedies. And consumers can only look to practitioners for guidance.

New information technologies are being brought online to provide distributors, consumers, and practitioners fair and accurate information about the appropriate use of dietary supplements. The Informatics Institute for Complementary and Integrative Medicine in Bethesda, Maryland (www.iicim.com), the TAI Sophia Institute in Columbia, Maryland, the University of Exeter in the United Kingdom, and other sources are committed to developing accessible databases on dietary supplements for professional reference in the practice of integrative medicine.

MEDICAL EDUCATION

The issues considered thus far point to the clear need for enhanced and improved education at the medical school, postgraduate medical, and continuing medical education (CME) levels. CME programs are met with the challenge that current practitioners have generally had no exposure in medical school or in postgraduate medical training. According to surveys conducted by the Center for Research in Medical Education at Thomas Jefferson University, as cited in chapter 1, the majority of today's medical students in all graduation years and among all classes want more education in integrative medicine. The proportion is increasing with each graduating year. Among classes in medical school, the proportion is relatively high in the first year (when entering students carry the culture of the general population), declines somewhat in the second and third years (as students become professionalized and generally witness little reinforcement for the teaching of integrative medicine), and rises again in the fourth year (after students have been exposed to the problems and questions of patients).

Much curriculum development and faculty development remains to be done in this area, and the traditional support of state and federal governments for medical education and training could be well utilized to help provide medical schools with the needed resources and incentives. In the interim, it is incumbent on providers of health care services to help stimulate appropriate CME and in-service training for health professions staffs so that practitioners may be knowledgeable and helpful to their patients in seeking guidance on the use of integrative medicine.

PUBLIC POLICY ISSUES

State governments have developed a traditional role in regulating medical practice and in helping support medical education. The federal government maintains a unique and critical role in stimulating and supporting medical research, regulating medical products and devices, protecting the public health, helping build health care infrastructure, and is now paying one-third of the costs of health care in America. Policy makers at the state and federal levels should become more knowledgeable about the needs and opportunities relative to integrative medicine.

The bipartisan Congressional Caucus on Complementary and Alternative Medicine and Dietary Supplements was organized to help serve this purpose, cochaired in the Senate by Sen. Tom Harkin (D-Iowa) and Sen. Orrin Hatch (R-Utah) and in the House of Representatives by Rep. Dennis Kucinich (D-Ohio) and Rep. Dan Burton (R-Indiana), who has also chaired the Committee on Government Reform Committee and its Subcommittee on Health and Human Rights. In 2007, it appears that there will be a new House Caucus on Dietary Supplements co-chaired by Reps. Chris Cannon (R-Utah) and Frank Pallone (D-NJ).

Some voluntary professional groups are beginning to work with members of the caucus and other elected representatives to broaden and deepen federal support for appropriate analyses and programs in integrative medicine. The regulatory legislation governing dietary supplements has not changed since the Dietary Supplement Health and Education Act of 1994 (but see previous paragraph).

Although funding for the National Center for Complementary and Alternative Medicine had increased each year since it was mandated by Congress in 1992, until the current budget cycle, it is critical that other federal agencies charged with programs relative to health resources and services, primary care, health professions training and workforce development, consumer education, health services research, and other areas be brought to bear on the important challenge and opportunity of integrative medicine. Integrative medicine has an important role that requires further articulation in Congressional actions on medical liability insurance reform and the national patient safety and quality assurance initiative.

Public support together with private innovation, and respect for the art and science of traditions of medical practice, have been the hallmarks for medical advancement and should continue to be the case for integrative medicine.

RESOURCES

Many individual and professional groups work with members of these caucuses and organizations to broaden and deepen federal support for programs on dietary supplements and integrative medicine.

The Congressional Caucus on Complementary and Alternative
  Medicine (CAM) and Dietary Supplements
  http://reform.house.gov/WHR/Hearings

Senate cochairmen
Sen. Tom Harkin (D-Iowa, www.harkin.senate.gov)
Sen. Orrin Hatch (R-Utah, www.hatch.senate.gov),

House cochairmen
Rep. Dan Burton (R-Indiana, www.house.gov/burton)
Rep. Dennis Kucinich (D-Ohio, www.kucinich.house.gov)

The mission of the caucus is to offer an opportunity for members of
Congress to learn about the growing role of complementary and alternative health practices and natural foods in improving the health and well-
being of millions of Americans. The CAM caucus runs seminars on policy
issues, on specific therapies, and on advances in research.

Office of Dietary Supplements (ODS)
National Institutes of Health
U.S. Department of Health and Human Services
http://dietary-supplements.info.nih.gov
Director: Paul M. Coates, PhD

The mission of ODS is to strengthen knowledge and understanding of
dietary supplements by evaluating scientific information, stimulating and
supporting research, disseminating research results, and educating the
public to foster an enhanced quality of life and health.

The National Center for Complementary and Alternative Medicine
  (NCCAM)
National Institutes of Health
U.S. Department of Health and Human Services
http://nccam.nih.gov/
Acting Director: Margaret Chesney, MD

NCCAM is dedicated to exploring complementary and alternative
healing practices in the context of rigorous science, training CAM researchers, and disseminating authoritative information to the public and
professionals.

Some General Guidelines for the Use of Herbal Medicines

- The clinician should take a careful history of the patient's use of herbs and other supplements.
- An accurate medical diagnosis must be made before using herbs for symptomatic treatment.
- *Natural* is not necessarily *safe*: Attention should be paid to quality of product, dosage, and potential adverse effects, including interactions.
- Herbal treatments should, for the most part, be avoided in pregnancy (and contemplated pregnancy) and lactation.
- Herbal usage in children should be done with care, using the appropriate dosage based on weight.
- Adverse effects should be recorded, and dosage reduced or the product discontinued. It can be carefully restarted to ascertain whether it is the source of the problem.
- Manufacturer should use GMP standards and be certified by a third party, such as National Nutritional Foods Association (NNFA) and United States Pharmacopoeia (USP).

CHAPTER 10

Future Health Care

Navigating Ongoing
Institutional Politics

Although many people, including physicians, are turning to CAM—using it, exploring it, becoming interested in seeing what it can and cannot do—the field is still in a tenuous position vis-à-vis conventional medicine. Physicians remain guarded in recommending CAM to their patients, and patients continue to refrain from discussing their use of CAM with their physicians.[227] One of the main routes toward legitimacy for CAM is research. However, because single studies require confirmation through replication, it may be years before conclusive findings appear. Integrative health care centers (IHCs) are a second route toward legitimacy, representing the experiential side of clinical testing. However, since IHCs are so new, we still do not know whether they, as a generic mechanism of delivering integrative health care, are equipped to accept this burden.

Some of the centers in our study are showing that they are able and willing to meet the challenge. But others are faltering, programmatically, financially, or both. Are these successes and problems inherent to the structure of IHCs or particular to the individual centers? We try to answer this question by systematizing our findings. We present what we believe, based on our research, are the main factors behind both the strengths and weaknesses of the centers in our study.

Financial support. The more successful centers have several sources of financial support. Even centers with generous donors (from either benefactors or the medical center) are constantly searching for and developing additional sources of revenue. Some of these, such as yoga classes, relate specifically to the clinic. Others pertain to the broader activities of the center, such as retreats or courses with registration fees that offer continuing education. Most importantly, research grants are essential, not only because of the academic setting but in general as a revenue enhancer. Research has the added benefit of fostering support from the wider medical community and furthering the legitimacy of integrative health care.

Support from the medical community. Centers must foster positive and strong working and personal relations with their relevant medical community. In the more successful centers in our study, directors have taken the time to build personal relations and trust with hospital physicians. Besides direct communication, engaging in joint research projects offers a vehicle toward acceptance. In a few centers, research is a primary factor in choosing which therapies to offer, generally because hospital physicians are already engaged in or interested in researching certain therapies. Nevertheless, all center directors must be conversant with the research on a range of therapies to justify their choices and to gain the ear first and then the minds and hearts of physicians.

A clear mission. The meaning and practice of integration vary among the IHCs in our study. Although the more successful centers practice a highly organized form of integrative medicine, not all centers have the resources to pursue this form, especially not in their early stages of development. What is more important than the substance, we believe, is constructing a form of integration suitable to the capacity of the center and the culture of the relevant medical community. Also, clarity in presenting what the center does and seeks to accomplish helps to assuage any concerns that hospital (or other) physicians may harbor. We can differentiate three levels of integration based on the practices in the centers we studied.

1. At a low end, patients who self-refer integrate themselves. Alternatively, as one director said, practitioners who do more than one therapy integrate themselves. This type of integration is the least satisfactory to all concerned. If centers are practicing in this manner, they would best be served by working to develop a tighter model.

2. At a middle level, someone at the center, either the director or a staff nurse or the first practitioner that a patient sees, functions as an integrative consultant. These individuals coordinate the care of patients who see more than one practitioner; make decisions, together with the patient, about sequencing and longevity of treatment; and inform practitioners as well as physicians outside the center about the care patients are receiving. Some centers select a practitioner or physician to be a team manager and function as an integrator, especially for patients who see more than one practitioner or whose care requires that practitioners coordinate or consult with physicians. Other clinics have developed team managers for each type of therapy offered by the clinic. We found that

this middle level of integration is not a function of center size or resources. It develops after careful thought about the notion of integration
and ability of the center to commit to the practice of integration.

3. At a high end, integration includes both someone functioning as
an "integrative consultant" as well as regular interactions, both informal
and formal, among practitioners and physicians. Directors in centers with
more resources and capacity structure systematic interactions in weekly
or monthly case conferences or didactic meetings. The major problem
that arises with regularly scheduled meetings is forgone fees. Many centers pay their fee-for-service practitioners to attend case conference meetings. Others combine salary and fee-for-service arrangements to allow for
interaction. In some centers it may be useful to invite hospital physicians
to these sessions.

A clear approach to quality assurance. The centers in our study vary
in their standards of quality assurance, making the weaker ones vulnerable to criticism from the medical profession. Two practices in particular
stand out. Because qualification standards for practitioners are geo-
graphically diverse, center directors need to be transparent about their
criteria for selection and the institutional scope of practice for each practitioner. Some of the directors in our study did a considerable amount
of prior investigation about practitioner standards and worked with
the hospital's legal counsel to set criteria down on paper. One possible
shortcoming that may entail issues of risk management is the irregularity
with which MDs sign off on the medical charts and treatment plans.[228]
Whether or not hospitals require surveys, it is a good idea to conduct
these as frequently as possible, both to monitor needs, demands, short-
comings, and progress, as well as to gather ammunition for going to the
administration with requests.

*Rational policies and procedures to address credentialing, liability,
and other legal concerns.* Credentialing schemes have been innovative in
the early, start-up years of IHCs as enterprising clinicians and administrators have turned to existing models within conventional care for mechanisms to get CAM services accepted within their institutions. In terms
of liability issues, though, many if not most IHCs have been addressing
legal issues on an ad hoc basis, either ignoring liability concerns on one
hand, or slavishly adhering to overly rigid dictates from hospital legal
counsel on the other. Rational frameworks now exist in the literature
to address liability issues and integrate liability concerns into clinical decision making; IHCs in the future are well advised to avail themselves
of these frameworks so as to rationalize policies that optimize the best
features of integrative care while maintains concerns for minimizing liability risk.

Although there is no single, reproducible model for integrative care in the United States, the foregoing points illustrate some of the major factors that to date have made existing IHCs viable. These factors, in addition to the strategies outlined throughout the book, are likely to help IHCs of the future successfully navigate new obstacles and challenges.

Conclusion

Integrative health care is an emerging phenomenon in the United States. Its contours are still being defined as different integrative health care centers (IHCs) emerge with idiosyncratic and novel formats within U.S. hospitals and health care systems. This study reviews some of the shared ground—and dissonance—among leading institutions grappling with funding and ongoing financing; institutional acceptance and growth; credentialing issues; malpractice liability risk management; and dietary supplement policies in their integrative health care centers and affiliated institutions.

In tackling these issues, the IHCs are helping to bridge medical research and evaluation of CAM therapies, standards of education and training established by professional organizations, and legislative and judicial recognition of CAM practitioners (which occurs largely through licensure and malpractice rules, respectively). In the long run, the success of integrative health care, as an evolution over the historical opposition of biomedical care to CAM therapies, rests in large part on the extent to which proponents of integrative centers will succeed in overcoming institutional barriers to achieve a new vision of health and health care. Such success, in turn, depends on a combination of legal and legislative, medical, and sociological factors.

Concepts and models of integrative care are evolving as clinical caregivers and institutions from different ranks begin to see beyond healing the split between conventional medicine and CAM therapies. These models move toward a comprehensive system of health care that incorporates a range of healing modalities from our global historical heritage and common cultural patrimony. They move along a spectrum from physiological, to emotional, to spiritual, with each layer assimilating aspects of the others. Such a spectrum of comprehensive care has been analogized to

Abraham Maslow's hierarchy of needs, in which some human needs (e.g., esteem) come into the foreground as other needs are met (e.g., survival).[229]

On an institutional level, there is a saying circulating among leaders of these centers at conferences and policy gatherings: "If you've seen one integrative health care center, you've seen one integrative health care center."[230] The humor and wisdom of this sentiment lies in the evolving experiment—the fact that although the centers share a commitment to integrating conventional and CAM therapies in conventional medical settings, each center has different sources of support, faces unique obstacles, and overcomes institutional (and legal) barriers in individual ways.

Those who are pioneers of integrative care within larger health care institutions each have a different story to tell. Collectively, they share common struggles and strategies around legal and liability issues, yet clearly tailor their efforts to the politics of individual institutions, to the vagaries of individual state statutes and administrative and judicial decisions, and to the desires and visions of individual leaders, funders, and players with strong egos and personalities. In assessing the emergence of integrative care, and in telling the story of its early unfolding, we canvassed both a significant group of the university-based centers and the significant players within each center. Due to the availability of various personnel (and the fact that they do not get paid for these interviews), most of our telephone sessions were with medical directors and administrators of integrative health care centers; less frequently, we were able to interview hospital legal counsel and pharmacists; finally, we also interviewed some practitioners.

From the perspective of this first group—medical directors and administrators—the hurdles may appear more numerous and larger than from the perspective of the CAM practitioners themselves. But comments from one CAM practitioner, an acupuncturist, within the second group—the CAM professionals involved in integration—provide the flavor of excitement expressed by those historically outside the medical system, now finding opportunities to work within it:

> I was honored to get the call. When I got here I was inundated with information—it was great to see how the institution has endorsed so many holistic and alternative modalities for cancer care. They have so many programs for patients and families members (such as Tai Chi, Tibetan medicine). There is so much dovetailing with other . . . [similar] centers; we can share visits and information among centers.

A massage therapist emphasized the ability to work in a multidisciplinary clinical team in a medical setting:

Having gone from private/fee-for-service to contract to being salaried on the staff, I feel more a part of the team; making more of a difference than individually, working with nurses and doctors.

The acupuncturist echoed the theme of team building, but emphasized the fact that these teams are tackling different modalities than one normally experiences in U.S. hospitals:

In hospital settings they see a lot of doctors, nurses, respiratory therapists and we're a different group. We represent that integrative healing model but we wear regular clothes, not lab clothes. We have to explain who we are, what we do. This whole program is synergistically involved with the medical aspect of healing: Integrative medicine is the new medicine that all doctors will need to go through, bringing together all the therapies we see around the world.

This last statement succinctly articulates the goal of medical pluralism that in important part undergirds ideals of integrative medicine—the bringing together of therapies represented globally, including other healing traditions, within the conventional health care setting. By crafting policies and strategies to address institutional politics, social and cultural issues, and legal issues in the domains of credentialing, liability management, and dietary supplements, the sample centers are forging new models of health care, and in so doing, overcoming legal and social barriers to integrative health.

Inclusion of CAM therapies and practitioners in the diagnostic and therapeutic regimens of conventional caregivers may remain complicated and controversial for some time. Given the individual stamp of each integrative center, the diversity of CAM practitioners, and the extent to which relevant law varies by state and provider, it may be difficult to emerge with national models for integrative care. Nonetheless, the pioneering efforts described in this book offer potential roadmaps as other clinical centers around the country explore the attempt to bridge conventional and CAM therapies, and thus to bring the best of both to patient care.

APPENDIX A

Interview Questions
(Policies and Procedures)

1. **Background and Credentialing**

   1.1 Does the clinic have a formal relationship with a hospital or medical school? Which one? What is the type of affiliation? Who at the clinic reports to whom within a hospital medical school?

   1.2 Who initiated the clinic? What kind of funding was provided for this (e.g., percentage donated and from what sources)? Is the clinic financially viable and self-sustaining?

   1.3 What are the types of clinical service providers (MD providers; non-MD providers and type)?

   1.4 What are the top 10 (or fewer) services offered (from most to least utilized and percentage)?

   1.5 Discuss credentialing versus privileging—does institution perceive any legal and/or practical implications to granting or not granting hospital privileges to would-be providers? For example, to what extent will this affect institution's ability to hire and fire providers, the liability of the affiliated hospital, and independence of the providers to practice CAM modalities?

   1.6 Compare credentialing of CAM practitioners to that of allied health professionals—is it more or less rigorous? What additional limitations are placed on CAM practitioners? To what extent do these additional limitations reflect statutory, scope of practice boundaries; internal institutional rules; or perceptions within the institution about the limits of specific provider's competence, safety issues, or concerns about collaborative practices between CAM and conventional providers?

1.7   What degree of MD supervision, if any, is required for each set of CAM practitioners? To what extent is such supervision mandated by statute, required by internal, pre-existing institutional rules applicable to allied health providers, or the result of changing internal perceptions concerning the reliability and safety of specific CAM practitioners?

1.8   Are there any institutional training requirements specific to CAM practitioners? Does the institution have a plan for educating CAM practitioners to deepen their understanding of medical realities; to what extent does the clinic plan to educate physicians and allied health providers in CAM theories and practices, and thus bridge the communication gap between two sets of providers?

2. Liability (including informed consent)

2.1   To what extent do patients self-refer versus come through MD versus CAM practitioner's referrals (percentage)?

2.2   How is the clinic integrated with conventional medical services? What barriers and challenges arise, particularly where there are overlapping scopes of practice between providers?

2.3   What is the intake procedure and who performs the intake and/or writes treatment plan?

2.4   What are the top 10 conditions treated (list from most to least and percentage)?

2.5   Does the clinic work with a CAM practitioner network for outside referrals?

2.6   Does the clinic provide any inpatient services? Which ones?

2.7   To what extent are providers engaged in joint treatment or share treatment plans? How are discussions handled for such treatment plans? Who has the authority to trump whom in these discussions?

2.8   What documentation is required to limit potential liability? What documentation is recommended? To what extent do policies or suggestions arise from state laws, rules from regulatory boards, internal institutional requirements, or judgments by clinic directors?

2.9   How is the duty to refer handled—does the clinic impose any requirements on CAM practitioners in this regard? Do physicians have any obligation to refer their patients to their CAM practitioner counterparts within the clinic?

2.10   Are any scripts provided for informed consent? How might they differ for different types of providers and therapies?

2.11   Whether or not the center has a policy concerning informed consent, how do providers handle conversations and inform patients regarding risks and benefits for combinations of therapies (i.e., conventional and CAM) when there is little evidence base for even understanding such risks and benefits?

2.12   Are there any other ways in which the clinic attempts to limit its liability exposure? Does the hospital have any similar or different approaches?

2.13   To what extent do common-law rules within the state regarding assumption of risk affect the way that clinical care is delivered—e.g., whether the patient can make a choice, must sign a carefully drafted form, and/or must verbally indicate responsibility for choosing a therapeutic option involving CAM therapies?

3. Dietary Supplements

3.1   Does the clinic have any policy regarding provision of (or counseling regarding) dietary supplements? If not, are there any informal understandings?

3.2   Are such policy and/or informal understandings within the clinic consistent or inconsistent with those of the affiliated hospital? What rationale is given for discrepancies?

3.3   If the institution lacks a coherent policy regarding provision of dietary supplements, how do individual practitioners (both conventional and CAM practitioners) handle patient inquiries regarding supplements?

3.4   What are the providers' beliefs and practices with patients regarding supplements?

3.5   Are there formal processes for reporting adverse events?

3.6   What provisions are made for documentation?

3.7   To what extent does the clinic support or discourage use of dietary supplements as part of an overall treatment plan?

3.8   Does the institution's position depend on evidence-based practices, and how does the institution reconcile such a position with the ability of acupuncturists to dispense Chinese herbs within their legally authorized scope of practice?

3.9   What role does the clinic ascribe to patient choices and preferences as opposed to the physician's obligation, particularly in the area of dietary supplements, to do no harm?

List of Centers Interviewed

Medical School of University (if applicable)	Name of Center/Hospital
Albert Einstein Medical College	Continuum Center for Health and Healing, Beth Israel Hospital
Columbia University	Columbia Integrative Medicine Program
Cornell University	Cornell Center for Complementary and Integrative Medicine
Duke University	Duke Center for Integrative Medicine
George Washington University	George Washington University Center for Integrative Medicine
Mayo Clinic	Complementary and Integrative Medicine Program
Medical University of South Carolina	Closed
Memorial Sloan Kettering	Integrative Medicine Service Program
Oregon Health Sciences University	Oregon Center for Complementary and Alternative Medicine in Neurological Disorders
Stanford University School of Medicine	Stanford Center for Integrative Medicine

Medical School of University (if applicable)	Name of Center/Hospital
Stonybrook University	Wellness Program, University Center for CAM, Stonybrook University Hospital
University of Arizona School of Medicine	Program in Integrative Medicine
University of California, San Francisco	Osher Center for Integrative Medicine
University of Colorado	University of Colorado Hospital
University of Maryland	Center for Integrative Medicine
University of Medicine and Dentistry of New Jersey	Institute for Complementary and Alternative Medicine
University of Michigan	University of Michigan Integrative Medicine, Department of Family Medicine, University of Michigan Health System
University of Minnesota	Center for Spirituality and Healing
University of New Mexico	Section of Integrative Medicine, University of New Mexico Health Sciences Center
University of North Carolina at Chapel Hill	Program on Integrative Medicine
University of Pennsylvania	Penn Therapy & Fitness Science Center
University of Pittsburgh, Shadyside	Center for Complementary Medicines
University of Texas MD Anderson Cancer Center	Integrative Medicine Program Place of Wellness
Yale University	Yale-Griffin Hospital Institute for Health and Healing
—	California Pacific Medical Center
—	St. Barnabas Medical Center

Clinic Characteristics

The following figures are all percentages of respondents. The figures in each category may not add to 100 due to rounding. Where 100 appears, it represents the percentage of those offering the treatment, not of all respondents.

Financial Structure

Initial Donor Contribution

Large	26
Medium	7
Small	43
None	22

Fund-raising

Major	26
Minor	65
None	17

Accepts insurance	57
Most patients pay out of pocket	78

Practitioners

Fee-for-service only	61
Salary only	17
Mixed salary and fee-for-service	22

Financial security
    Confident   65
    Concerned   7
    Uncertain   26
    Have or planning independent status   13

Administrative Structure

Medical director   87
Operative
    Less than 2 years   30
    2–5 years   35
    More than 5 years   43
Less than 5 practitioners   35
5–10 practitioners   22
10–15 practitioners   17
More than 15 practitioners   30
Practitioners
    Mostly part-time   57
    Mostly full-time   7
    Mixed   35
Outpatient only   65
    Expect to expand to include inpatient   52
Inpatient only   4
    Expect to expand to include outpatient   0
Both outpatient and inpatient   30

Delivery of Care

Proportion of patients with physician referral
    Less than one-quarter   35
    One-quarter to one-half   39
    Over one-half   26
    Referral required   22
Primary care physician required   43
Primary care at clinic   13

Initial screening by nurse	17
Initial approval by medical director	48
No formal triage	39
Informed consent before invasive treatment	100
Refer to practitioners in community	43
Offers	
Acupuncture	87
Massage	83
Mind–body	87
Movement	61
Physical therapy	61
Nutritional counseling	70
Herbal counseling	65
Chiropractic	30
Homeopathy	30

Working Relations

Supportive hospital administration	65
Regular staff meetings	78
MD supervision	
Random	78
Systematic	30
Close liaisons with outside physicians	83
Regular contact with MDs in hospital	83
Informational (grand rounds)	87
Active networking	78
Research ties	78
Progress in raising physician interest	
High	61
Medium	7
Low	30

APPENDIX D

Guidelines for Dietary Supplements

GENERAL CONSIDERATIONS FOR THE USE OF HERBS

Changes in the practice of medicine are causing a shift to increasing self-care with more benign, less invasive treatments. Therefore, it is critical that practicing clinicians (and, in turn, patients) be made aware of the indications, actions, and drug interactions of herbal remedies.

The World Health Organization estimates that 80% of the world's population relies on herbal medicine. Meanwhile, the use of herbs in the United States is expanding rapidly, to the point where herbal products are readily found in most pharmacies and supermarkets. From 1990 to 1997, as the use of complementary/alternative medicine rose from 34% to 42%, herbal use quadrupled from 3% to 12% (Eisenberg et al., note 2).

It is worth remembering that these rapid changes have come by popular demand. The public has discovered that natural medicines often provide a safe, effective, and economical alternative, and research is increasingly validating this finding. Many of those who use herbal and high-dose vitamin products fail to tell their physicians. Either they assume so-called natural products are harmless and not worth mentioning or they fear telling health professionals who may be skeptical about their use. However, health professionals are beginning to familiarize themselves with the subject. Aside from some advantages of natural products, herb–drug interactions are a growing concern: Almost one in five prescription drug users are also using supplements (Eisenberg et al., note 2).

In Europe, there is less of a problem because herbs are classified with other pharmaceutical products and routinely prescribed by doctors. In fact, in Germany prescriptions of St John's wort (SJW) outnumber those for all other antidepressants. Most of the research to date is European, because the natural products industry has had the financial incentive to do the necessary research. The United States has recently joined in these efforts and the National Institutes of Health (NIH) National Center for Complementary and Alternative Medicine and the National Institute of Mental Health (NIMH) completed a $4.3 million joint clinical trial to determine the efficacy of St John's wort in major depression. Herbal studies are now in progress at a number of major U.S. medical universities.

Herbs for Health

In the Eisenberg survey, two of the top five conditions for which consumers sought alternative treatment were anxiety and depression. Besides SJW, there are other popular herbs for these and related problems: kava for relief of stress and anxiety (until recent concerns about potential effects on the liver), ginkgo biloba for senile dementia or benign forgetfulness, and valerian for sleep.

Many current drugs are derived from plants. Common examples are morphine from the opium poppy, digitalis from foxglove, and reserpine from rauwolfia (Indian snakeroot). In many cases, pharmaceuticals remain the treatment of choice. However, when appropriate, herbs may be preferred for the following reasons:

- Herbs are generally less likely to cause side effects. When they do occur, they are generally milder. In fact, in the absence of side effects, patients often do not notice the subtle improvements that occur as these natural medicines begin to take effect. This contrasting lack of side of effects may also confound double blind studies. A partial explanation for the milder side effects may be that the original plant constituents are more compatible with metabolism and body chemistry.
- Although the isolated active ingredient has been assumed to be most effective, there are advantages to using the whole plant.
- These combinations may also yield a variety of effects. For example, by its action on the brain, kava acts as an anxiety reliever, while its relaxant effects are due to its direct action on both smooth and striated muscle.
- Herbs are working physiologically to restore balance rather than simply targeting a symptom. As a result, herbs often tend to take effect more gradually than pharmaceuticals.

Safety

Side effects of drugs can be serious, the worst being death by overdose. According to one report, overdoses yielded an annual rate of 30.1 deaths per one million prescriptions of antidepressant. To quote Norman Farnsworth, PhD, Professor of Pharmacognosy at the University of Illinois, Chicago: "Based on published reports, side effects or toxic reactions associated with herbal medicines in any form are rare. . . . In fact, of all classes of substances . . . to cause toxicities of sufficient magnitude to be reported in the United States, plants are the least problematic." (pers. commun.) It is important to caution patients that if they feel any ill effects from an herbal product, they should inform the prescribing doctor. Then, depending on the severity, the patient should either reduce the dose or stop taking the herb altogether. Unlike pharmaceuticals, withdrawal reactions are rarely an issue.

It is essential to obtain a complete drug and herbal history. There are contraindicated combinations, which should be covered individually; however, many combinations work well together. For example, individuals taking a drug that is metabolized by the liver can be protected by the liver-supporting herb, milk thistle (*Silybum marianum*).

Pregnancy, Breastfeeding, and Children

Many herbs have not been approved for use by pregnant and nursing women in the guidelines of the German Commission E, the equivalent of the U.S. Food and Drug Administration (FDA). Now available in English translation, the German Commission E has published a collection of reports based on safety and efficacy data on more than 200 herbs.

Herbs may often be a treatment of choice for children. Despite lack of modern research, centuries of use have shown many products to be safe when dosed appropriately by weight.

Aging

Considering the phenomenon of polypharmacy in the elderly and problems of impaired metabolism and clearance, herbs may offer an alternative to drugs. However, we must be aware of herb–drug interactions. SJW can be very useful for depression in the elderly, ginkgo for cognitive decline, and kava for sedation (but see section Herbs for Health), without the adverse effects of the benzodiazepines. These herbs can be used in combination with each other as well.

SELECTION AND USE OF HERBS

Standardized Extracts

For those new to the medicinal use of herbs, dose selection can be confusing. As discussed previously, unlike synthetic drugs containing a single compound, herbs often have a number of different active ingredients. Even these vary in proportion, based on many factors including where the plant was grown and when (season or even the time of day) it was harvested. Manufacturers may adjust the mixture to help account for these variations.

In order to standardize the product, that is, to have a consistent, measured amount of product per unit dose, one ingredient is selected as the marker, usually the presumed active ingredient. Though research may reveal different or additional active ingredients, for convenience the designated constituent usually remains the accepted marker. This situation is demonstrated in the example of St John's wort.

SJW is standardized to hypericin, the long-accepted active antidepressant ingredient. Further research has found hyperforin to be a likely active ingredient. Some SJW products are actually standardized for both. In any case, all compounds (even as-yet-undiscovered contributors) remain distributed throughout the plant, alongside the hypericin. As a result, the standardization of hypericin serves as a useful guidepost for the strength of *all* the (active) ingredients.

Hypericin content is listed on the label, with most products using a 0.3 percent concentration, so that a 300 mg capsule contains 0.9 mg (0.3 × 300 mg) of hypericin. In kava, the marker is kavalactones, and in ginkgo, flavone glycosides.

Herbal Preparations and Dosing

Herbs can be purchased as teas, tinctures, tablets, and capsules. Teas and tinctures, being liquid, are absorbed more rapidly, and with a shorter duration of action. Tinctures are made by soaking one part herbal material with 5 or 10 parts by weight of alcohol, making a 1:5 or 1:10 concentration. To remove the alcohol taste, the tincture can be placed in warm water or tea for a few minutes to let the alcohol evaporate. Glycerin may also be used instead of alcohol, but the resulting extract is weaker.

Capsules and tablets are the most common delivery system. Gelatin or vegetable-based capsules are filled with powdered dried herb, while tablets are powdered herbs, compressed into a solid pill, often with a variety of inert ingredients as fillers.

Tablets and capsules are supplied in a variety of sizes and strengths, so it is important to read the label carefully. The label also usually gives an average suggested dose as a guideline, based on research and clinical use. It is recommended to start at the low end, watch for a response, including unwanted effects, and adjust the dose accordingly. For example, some patients may do well on 300 mg of SJW once a day, while others need four times that dose. Most fall in the middle, with the recommended 300 mg three times daily. Some herbs, such as kava, take effect immediately, while others take days, weeks (SJW, ginkgo), or even months to do so, with individual variation.

REGULATORY ISSUES

Most herbal products are regulated as dietary supplements. In 1994, the U.S. Dietary Supplement Health and Education Act (known as DSHEA) set new guidelines with regard to quality, labeling, packaging, and marketing of supplements. It also sparked a surge of interest in herbal products. DSHEA allows manufacturers to make "statements of nutritional support for conventional vitamins and minerals." Since herbs are not nutritional in the conventional sense, DSHEA allows them to make only what they call "structure and function claims," but no therapeutic or prevention claims. Thus, an SJW label can claim that it "optimizes mood," but cannot say "natural antidepressant," which would be a therapeutic claim.

Because the labels (by law) give insufficient information, it is particularly important for the health practitioner to be well educated in this area. Ideally, supplements would be labeled so that the purchaser would know exact indications and possible side effects, as with over-the-counter (OTC) medicines.

Quality control is essential, with assurance that the product contains the ingredients and quantities as labeled, and without such contaminants as bacteria, molds, or pesticides. There are trade and professional organizations, such as the American Herbal Products Association (AHPA), that are setting standards called *good manufacturing practices* (GMP) for the herbal industry. In general, we recommend buying herbal products from a recognized manufacturer.

There are a number of excellent Web sites on the subject:

Alternative Medicine Foundation, Inc.: HerbMed.org
American Botanical Council: www.herbalgram.org
Herb Research Foundation: www.herbs.org
Natural Product Research Consultants (NPRC): www.nprc.com
The Natural Pharmacist: www.TNP.com

REFERENCES AND RESOURCES

Blumenthal, M., Goldberg, A., & Brinckmann, J. (2000). *Herbal medicine: Expanded commission E monographs.* Newton, MA: Integrative Medicine Communications.

Cott, J. M. (1997). In vitro receptor binding and enzyme inhibition by *Hypericum perforatum* extract. *Pharmacopsychiatry, 30*(Suppl. II), 108–112.

Davies, L. P., Drew, C. A., Duffield, P., Johnston, G. A., & Jamieson, D. D. (1992). Kava pyrones and resin: studies on GABAA, GABAB and benzodi-azepine binding sites in rodent brain. *Pharmacology & Toxicology, 71*(2), 120–126.

Dorn, M. (2000) [Efficacy and tolerability of Baldrian versus oxazepam in non-organic and non-psychiatric insomniacs: a randomised, double-blind, clinical, comparative study]. *Forsch Komplementarmed Klass Naturheilkd 7,* 79–84.

Eisenberg, D. M., Davis, R. B., Ettner, S. L., Appel, S., Wilkey, S., Van Rompay, M., & Kessler, R. C. (1998). Trends in alternative medicine use in the United States, 1990–1997: Results of a follow-up national survey. *Journal of the American Medical Association, 280,* 1569–1575.

European Scientific Cooperative on Phytotherapy Monographs on the Medicinal Use of Plants. (1997). Exeter, UK: ESCOP.

Fontana, R. J., Lown, K. S., Paine, M. F., Fortlage, L., Santella, R. M., Felton, J. S., Knize, M. G., Greenberg, A., & Watkins, P. B. (1999). Effects of a chargrilled meat diet on expression of CYP3A, CYP1A, and P-glycoprotein levels in healthy volunteers. *Gastroenterology, 117,* 89–98.

Fugh-Berman, A., & Cott, J. M. (1999). Dietary supplements and natural products as psychotherapeutic agents. *Psychosomatic Medicine, 61,* 712–728.

Garrett, B. J., Cheeke, P. R., Miranda, C. L., Goeger, D. E., & Buhler, D. R. (1982). Consumption of poisonous plants by rats. *Toxicology Letter, 10,* 183–188.

Hypericum Depression Trial Study Group. (2002). Effect of *Hypericum perforatum* (St John's wort) in major depressive disorder: a randomized controlled trial. *Journal of the American Medical Association, 287,* 1807–1814.

Johne, A., Brockmoller, J., Bauer, S., Maurer, A., Langheinrich, M., & Roots, I. (1999). Pharmacokinetic interaction of digoxin with an herbal extract from St John's wort (*Hypericum perforatum*). *Clinical Pharmacology & Therapeutics, 66,* 338–345.

Kinzler, E., Kromer, J., & Lehmann, E. (1991). Wirksamkeit eines Kava-Spezial-Extraktes bei Patienten mit Angst-, Spannungs-und Erregungszustanden nicht-psychotischer Genese. *Arzneim Forsch/Drug Research, 41,* 584–588.

Landes, P. (1998). Market report. *HerbalGram, 42,* 64–65.

Linde, K., Ramirez, G., Mulrow, C. D., Pauls, A., Weidenhammer, W., & Melchart, D. (1996). St. John's wort for depression—an overview and meta-analysis of randomized clinical trials. *British Medical Journal, 313,* 253–258.

Maurer, A., Johne, A., Bauer, S., Brockmöller, J., Donath, F., Roots, I., Langheinrich, M., & Hübner, W. D. (1999). Interaction of St. John's wort extract with phenprocoumon. *European Journal of Clinical Pharmacology, 55,* A22.

McGuffin, M., Hobbs, C., Upton, R., & Goldberg, A. (1997). *Botanical safety handbook.* Boca Raton, FL: CRC Press.

Müller, W. E., Rolli, M., Schäfer, C., & Hafner, U. (1997). Effects of Hypericum extract (LI 160) in biochemical models of antidepressant activity. *Pharmacopsychiatry, 30*(Suppl. II), 102–107.

Newall, C. A., Anderson, L. A., & Phillipson, J. D. (1996). *Herbal medicines: A guide for health-care professionals.* London: The Pharmaceutical Press, pp. 239–240.

Ohnishi, A., Matsuo, H., Yamada, S., Takanaga, H., Morimoto, S., Shoyama, Y., Ohtani, H., & Sawada, Y. (2000). Effect of furanocoumarin derivatives in grapefruit juice on the uptake of vinblastine by Caco-2 cells and on the activity of cytochrome P450 3A4. *British Journal of Pharmacology, 130,* 1369–1371.

Piscitelli, S. C., Burstein, A. H., Chaitt, D., Alfaro, R. M., & Falloon, J. (2000). Indinavir concentrations and St John's wort. *Lancet, 355*(9203), 547–548.

Ruschitzka, F., Meier, P. J., Turina, M., Luscher, T. F., & Noll, G. (2000). Acute heart transplant rejection due to Saint John's wort. *Lancet, 355,* 548–549.

Santos, M. S., Ferreira, F., Faro, C., Pires, E., Carvalho, A. P., Cunha, A. P., & Macedo, T. (1994). The amount of GABA present in aqueous extracts of valerian is sufficient to account for [3H]GABA release in synaptosomes. *Planta Medicina, 60,* 475–476.

Schelosky, L., Raffauf, C., Jendroska, K., & Poewe, W. (1995). Letter to the Editor. *Journal of Neurology, Neurosurgery & Psychiatry, 45,* 639–640.

Shelton, R. C., Keller, M. B., Gelenberg, A. et al. (2001). Effectiveness of St. John's wort in major depression: a randomized controlled trial. *Journal of the American Medical Association, 285,* 1978–1986.

Upton, R., Graff, A., Williamson, E., Bevill, A., Ertl, F., Reich, E., Martinez, M., Lange, M., Wang, W., & Barrett, M. (1999). American herbal pharmacopoeia and therapeutic compendium on valerian root: Analytical, quality control, and therapeutic monograph. Santa Cruz, CA: American Herbal Pharmacopoeia.

Upton, R., Graff, A., Williamson, E., Bunting, D., Gatherum, D. M., Walker, E. B., & Cott, J. (1997). American herbal pharmacopoeia and therapeutic compendium on St. John's wort *Hypericum perforatum*: Quality control, analytical and therapeutic monograph. *HerbalGram, 40*(Suppl), 1–32.

Vorbach, E. U. (1997). Efficacy and tolerability of St. John's wort extract LI 160 vs. imipramine in patients with severe depressive episodes according to ICD-10. *Pharmacopsychiatry, 30*(Suppl. 2), 81–85.

Welch, C. A. (1995). In D. A. Ciraulo, R. I. Shader, D. J. Greenblatt, & W. Creelman. (Eds.), *Drug interactions in psychiatry* (2nd ed., p. 399). Baltimore: Williams & Wilkins.

Wichtl, M. (1994). In N. G. Bisset & M. Wichtl (Eds.), *Herbal drugs and phytopharmaceuticals: A handbook for practice on a scientific basis* (273–275). Boca Raton, FL: CRC Press.

Wolfman, C., Viola, H., Paladini, A., Dajas, F., & Medina, J. H. (1994). Possible anxiolytic effects of chrysin, a central benzodiazepine receptor ligand isolated from *Passiflora coerulea. Pharmacology, Biochemistry & Behavior, 47*(1), 1–4.

Yue, Q-Y., Bergquist, C., & Gerdén, B. (2000). Safety of St John's wort (*Hypericum perforatum*). *Lancet, 355,* 576–577.

Resources

Journals and Miscellaneous

Adams, K. E., Cohen, M. H., Jonsen, A. R., & Eisenberg, D. M. (2002). Ethical considerations of complementary and alternative medical therapies in conventional medical settings. *Annals of Internal Medicine, 137,* 660–664.

Cohen, M. H. (2003). Regulation, religious experience, and epilepsy: A lens on complementary therapies. *Epilepsy Behavior, 4,* 602–606.

Cohen, M. H. (2003). Complementary and integrative medical therapies, the FDA, and the NIH: Definitions and regulation. *Dermatology Therapy, 16,* 77–84.

Cohen, M. H. (2004). Healing at the borderland of medicine and religion: Regulating potential abuse of authority by spiritual healers. *Journal of Law & Religion, 18,* 373–426.

Cohen, M. H., & Eisenberg, D. M. (2002). Potential physician malpractice liability associated with complementary/integrative medical therapies. *Annals of Internal Medicine, 136,* 596–603.

Cohen, M. H., & Ruggie, M. (2004). Integrating complementary and alternative medical therapies in conventional medical settings: Legal quandaries and potential policy models. *Cincinnati Law Review, 72,* 671–729.

Cohen, M., & Schacter, S. (2004). Facilitating IRB consideration of protocols involving complementary and alternative medical therapies. *Clinical Researcher, 4,* 2–6.

Dietary Supplements Health Education Act, 103 P.L. 417; 108 Stat. 4325; 1994.

Dumoff, A. (1995). Malpractice liability of alternative/complementary health care providers: A view from the trenches. *Alternative and Complementary Therapies, 1,* 248; *Alternative and Complementary Therapies, 1,* 333.

Dumoff, A. (2002). Coding system for alternative and complementary therapies: It's not as easy as ABC. *Alternative and Complementary Therapies, 8,* 246.

Dumoff, A. (2000). Medical board prohibitions against physician supplements sales. *Alternative and Complementary Therapies, 6,* 226.

Dumoff, A. (2000). Regulating professional relationships: Kickback and self-referral restrictions on collaborative practice. *Alternative and Complementary Therapies, 6,* 41.

Dumoff, A. (1997). Understanding the Kassenbaum-Kennedy Health Care Act: Addressing legitimate concerns and irrational fears. *Alternative and Complementary Therapies, 3,* 309.

Dumoff, A. (1997). Legislation versus self-regulation in the somatic practices field: Comments from the Editor, *Alternative and Complementary Therapies, 3,* 220.

White House Commission on Complementary and Alternative Medicine Policy. (2002). Executive Summary, Final Report.

Ernst, E. E., & Cohen, M. H. (2001). Informed consent in complementary and alternative medicine. *Archives of Internal Medicine, 161,* 2288–2292.

Eisenberg, D. M., Cohen, M. H., Hrbek, A., Grayzel, J., van Rompay, M. I., & Cooper, R. A. (2002). Credentialing complementary and alternative medical providers. *Annals of Internal Medicine, 136,* 660–664.

Eisenberg, D. M. (1997). Advising patients who seek alternative medical therapies. *Annals of Internal Medicine, 127,* 61–69.

Federation of State Medical Boards. (2002). *Guidelines for complementary and alternative therapies in medical practice.* Available at www.fsmb.org

Federal Trade Commission. (2006). *Dietary supplements: An advertising guide for industry.* Available at www.ftc.gov

Food and Drug Administration Regulations on Statements Made for Dietary Supplements Concerning the Effect of the Product on the Structure or Function of the Body, 21 C.F.R. Part 101, 65:4 Fed. Reg. 1000 (Jan. 6, 2000).

Hathcock, J. (2001). Dietary supplements: How they are used and regulated. *Journal of Nutrition, 131,* 1114S–1117S.

Kaptchuk, T. J. (2001). Varieties of healing 1: Medical pluralism in the United States. *Annals of Internal Medicine, 135,* 189.

Kaptchuk, T. J. (2001). Varieties of healing 2: A taxonomy of unconventional healing practices, *Annals of Internal Medicine, 135,* 196.

Kemper, K., & Cohen, M. H. (2004). Ethics in complementary medicine: New light on old principles. *Contemporary Pediatrics, 21,* 61–72.

Marcus, D. M., & Grollman A. P. (2002). Botanical medicines—The need for new regulations. *New England Journal of Medicine, 347*), 2073.

McNamara, S. H. (2000). Regulation of dietary supplements. *New England Journal of Medicine, 343,* 1270.

Studdert, D. M., Eisenberg, D. M., Miller, F. H., Curto, D. A., Kaptchuk, T. J., & Brennan, T. A. (1998). Medical malpractice implications of alternative medicine [see comments]. *Journal of the American Medical Association, 280,* 1610.

Young, A. L., & Bass, I. S. (1995). The Dietary Supplement Health and Education Act. *Food & Drug Law Journal, 50,* 285–292.

Books

Callahan, Daniel. (Ed.). (2002). *The role of complementary and alternative medicine: Accommodating pluralism.* Georgetown University Press. Washington, DC.

Cohen, M. H. (1998). *Complementary and alternative medicine: Legal boundaries and regulatory perspectives.* Baltimore: Johns Hopkins University Press.

Cohen, M. H. (2000). *Beyond complementary medicine: Legal and ethical perspectives on health care and human evolution.* Ann Arbor, MI: University of Michigan Press.

Cohen, M. H. (2003). *Future medicine: Ethical dilemmas, regulatory challenges, and therapeutic pathways to health and human healing in human transformation.* Ann Arbor, MI: University of Michigan Press.

Faas, N. (Ed.). (2001). *Integrating complementary medicine into health systems: Benefits of complementary medicine.* Boulder, MD: Aspen Press.

Humber, J. M., & Almeder, R. F. (Eds.). (1998). *Alternative medicine and ethics.* Atlanta, GA: Humana Press.

Micozzi, M. S. (Ed.). (2006). *Fundamentals of complementary and alternative medicine* (3rd ed.). Philadelphia: Saunders-Elsevier.

Micozzi, M. S. (2007). *Complementary and integrative medicine in cancer care and prevention.* New York: Springer.

Slater, V., & Rankin-Box, D. (1996). *The nurses' handbook of complementary therapies.* New York: Churchill-Livingstone.

Notes

1. D. M. Eisenberg, R. C. Kessler, C. Foster, F. E. Norlock, D. R. Calkins, and T L. Delbanco, Unconventional medicine in the United States: Prevalence, costs, and patterns of use, *New England Journal of Medicine, 328*(4), 246–252 (1993).
2. D. M. Eisenberg, R. B. Davis, S. L. Ettner, S. Appel, S. Wilkey, M. Van Rompay, et al., Trends in alternative medicine use in the United States, 1990–1997: Results of a follow-up national survey, *Journal of the American Medical Association, 280*(18), 1569–1575 (1998).
3. Landmark Healthcare I. *The Landmark Report II on HMOs and Alternative Care.* Sacramento, CA: Landmark Healthcare, 1999.
4. B. M. Berman, The Cochrane Collaboration and evidence-based complementary medicine, *Journal of Alternative and Complementary Medicine, 3*(2), 191–194 (1997).
5. J. A. Astin, Why patients use alternative medicine: Results of a national study, *Journal of the American Medical Association, 279*(19), 1548–1553 (1998).
6. R. C. Kessler, R. B. Davis, D. F. Foster, M. I. Van Rompay, E. E. Walters, S. A. Wilkey, et al., Long-term trends in the use of complementary and alternative medical therapies in the United States, *Annals of Internal Medicine, 135*(4), 262–268 (2001).
7. R. B. Bausell, W. L. Lee, and B. M. Berman, Demographic and health-related correlates to visits to complementary and alternative medical providers, *Medical Care, 39*(2), 190–196 (2001).
8. B. G. Druss and R. A. Rosenheck, Association between use of unconventional therapies and conventional medical services. *Journal of the American Medical Association, 282*(7), 651–656 (1999).
9. J. Wooton and A. Sparber, Surveys of complementary and alternative medicine usage: Review of general population trends and specific populations, *Seminars in Integrative Medicine, 1*(1), 10–24 (2003).
10. P. M. Barnes et al., Complementary and alternative medicine use among adults: United States, 2002, *Seminars in Integrative Medicine, 2*(2), 54–70 (2004).

11. M. S. Micozzi, Complementary medicine: What is appropriate? Who will provide it?, *Annals of Internal Medicine, 129*, 65–66 (1998).
12. M. Ruggie, *Marginal to mainstream: Alternative medicine in America.* Cambridge: New York and London, 2004.
13. M. Ruggie and M. H. Cohen, Integrative medicine centers: Moving healthcare in a new direction, *Seminars in Integrative Medicine, 3*(1), 9–16 (2005).
14. P. M. Herman, B. M. Craig, and O. Caspi, Is complementary and alternative medicine (CAM) cost-effective? A systematic review, *BMC Complementary and Alternative Medicine, 5*(11), 1–15 (2005).
15. C. Hulme and A. F. Long, Square pegs and round holes? A review of economic evaluation of complementary and alternative medicine, *Journal of Alternative and Complementary Medicine, 11*(1), 179–188 (2005).
16. V. R. Kshettry et al., Complementary alternative medical therapies for heart surgery patients: Feasibility, safety and impact, *Journal of the Society of Thoracic Surgeons, 81*, 201–206 (2006).
17. H. M. Arthur, C. Patterson, and J. A. Stone, The role of complementary and alternative therapies in cardiac rehabilitation: A systematic review, *European Journal of Cardiovascular Prevention and Rehabilitation, 13*(1), 3–9 (2006).
18. K. V. Ergil, Chinese medicine. In M. S. Micozzi (ed.), *Fundamentals of complementary and integrative medicine* (3rd ed., pp. 375–417). New York and London: Elsevier, 2006.
19. M. S. Micozzi, *Fundamentals of complementary and integrative medicine,* 3rd ed. New York and London: Elsevier, 2006.
20. M. S. Micozzi, *Complementary and integrative medicine in cancer care and prevention.* New York: Springer, 2007.
21. D. J. Lawrence, B. Meeker, and M. S. Micozzi, *Best practices: Chiropractic management of low back pain.* American Public Health Association. Retrieved 2005 from http://apha.confex.com/apha/133am/chc/persons/edit.cgi
22. M. Hojat et al., Physician empathy in medical education and practice: Experience with the Jefferson Scale of Physician Empathy, *Seminars in Integrative Medicine, 1*(1), 25–40 (2003).
23. Significant progress has been made on related fronts, such as, for example, the work to develop and establish FDA regulations to govern good manufacturing practices (GMP's) for dietary supplements. Another looming issue is the development by the Codex Alimentarius Commission of international standards for dietary supplements. In July of 2005, the commission adopted the Guidelines for Vitamin and Mineral Food Supplements, triggering concern that the guidelines will restrict consumers' access "to the wide range of vitamin and mineral supplements of varying potencies legally sold in the United States. Others are concerned that the guidelines will limit the amount and type of information on the labels of dietary supplements sold in the United States. Still others believe that the guidelines will require dietary supplements to be sold as drugs in the United States." U.S. Food and Drug Administration, CFSAN/Office of Nutritional Products, Labeling and Dietary Supplements. "Responses to Questions about Codex and Dietary Supplements." Retrieved June 7, 2006 from http://www.cfsan.fda.gov/~dms/dscodex.html

24. Eisenberg et al., Trends, note 2.
25. American Hospital Association (Health Forum), *2000–2001 Complementary and Alternative Medicine Survey*. Chicago: American Hospital Association, 2002 (available at www.hospitalconnect.com).
26. M. H. Cohen, L. Sandler, A. Hrbek, R. B. Davis, and D. M. Eisenberg, Policies pertaining to complementary and alternative medical therapies in a random sample of 39 academic health centers, *Alternative Therapies in Health and Medicine, 11*(1), 36–40 (2005).
27. Anne Nedrow, Status of credentialing alternative providers within a subset of U.S. academic health centers, *Journal of Alternative and Complementary Medicine, 12*(3), 329–335 (2006).
28. F. McPherson and M. A. Schwenka, Use of complementary and alternative therapies among active duty soldiers, military retirees, and family members at a military hospital, *Military Medicine, 169,* 354–357 (May 2004).
29. P. Barnes, E. Powell-Griner, K. McFann, and R. Nahin. *Complementary and Alternative Medicine Use Among Adults: United States, 2002.* CDC Advance Data Report #343, May 27, 2004.
30. M. H. Cohen, Regulating 'healing': Notes on the ecology of awareness and the awareness of ecology, *St John's Law Review, 78*(4), 1167–1192 (2005).
31. *Report on Complementary and Alternative Medicine.* Washington, DC: National Academy of Sciences, 2005.
32. Michael H. Cohen, *Beyond complementary medicine: Legal and ethical perspectives on health care and human evolution* (Ann Arbor: University of Michigan Press, 2000); David M. Studdert, David M. Eisenberg, Francis H. Miller, D. A. Curto, Ted J. Kaptchuk, and Troyen A. Brennan, Medical malpractice implications of alternative medicine, *Journal of the American Medical Association, 280,* 1610 (1998) (describing malpractice liability of physicians for referrals to CAM providers).
33. Cohen (1998); Cohen, *Complementary and alternative medicine: Legal boundaries and regulatory perspectives*, at 9, pp. 1–180. Johns Hopkins University Press. Frontier legal issues, such as how to regulate touch in novel applications of mental health professions that dovetail with CAM modalities such as massage therapy and bodywork, remain largely unresolved. Michael H. Cohen, *Future medicine: Ethical dilemmas, regulatory challenges, and therapeutic pathways to health and healing in human transformation*, pp. 175–180. Ann Arbor: University of Michigan Press, 2003.
34. See, e.g., Phil B. Fontarosa and George D. Lundberg, Alternative medicine meets science, *Journal of the American Medical Association, 280,* 1618 (1998); Marcia Angell and Jerome P. Kassirer, Alternative medicine: The risks of untested and unregulated remedies, *New England Journal of Medicine, 339,* 839 (1998).
35. P. C. Walker, Evolution of a policy disallowing the use of alternative therapies in a health system, *American Journal of Health Policy, 57,* 1610–1990 (2000).
36. See, e.g., CA SB 577 (signed into law 9/23/02). The legislation provides that a person is not in violation of specified provisions of the Medical Practice Act that prohibit the practice of medicine without being licensed as a physician,

as long as the person does not engage in specified acts, and also makes specified disclosures to each client, which the client must acknowledge receipt of in writing. See also Minn. Stat. § 146A (allowing a broad range of CAM providers to offer services without requiring them to obtain licensure, but requiring them to register with a state agency that can receive consumer complaints); R.I. Gen. Laws § 23-74-1(3) (statute defines "unlicensed health care practices" as: "the broad domain of unlicensed healing methods and treatments, including, but not limited to: (i) acupressure; (ii) Alexander technique; (iii) aroma therapy; (iv) ayurveda; (v) cranial sacral therapy; (vi) crystal therapy; (vii) detoxification practices and therapies; (viii) energetic healing; (ix) rolfing; (x) Gerson therapy and colostrum therapy; (xi) therapeutic touch; (xii) herbology or herbalism; (xiii) polarity therapy; (xiv) homeopathy; (xv) nondiagnostic iridology; (xvi) body work; (xvii) reiki; (xviii) mind–body healing practices; (ixx) naturopathy; and (xx) Qi Gong energy healing").

37. White House Commission on Complementary and Alternative Medicine Policy, Final Report. (2002). Available at http://www.whccamp.hhs.gov/

38. David M. Eisenberg, Advising patients who seek alternative medical therapies, *Annals of Internal Medicine, 127,* 61 (1997) (arguing that physicians must abandon the policy of "don't ask and don't tell," and should make asking about use of CAM therapies a regular part of the medical interview).

39. Kaptchuk and Eisenberg, Varieties of medical pluralism I and II (2001), at 190, quoting Oliver Wendell Holmes, *Homeopathy and its kindred delusions.* Boston: W.D. Ticknor, 1842.

40. David M. Eisenberg, R. C. Kessler, C. Foster, F. E. Norlock, D. R. Calkin, and T. L. Delbanco, Unconventional medicine in the United States: Prevalence, costs, and patterns of use, *New England Journal of Medicine, 328,* 246, 256 (1993).

41. British Medical Association, *Complementary medicine: New approaches to good practice.* London: BMA, 1993.

42. National Center for Complementary and Alternative Medicine, *What Is Complementary and Alternative Medicine.* Available at http://nccam.nih .gov/health/whatiscam/#sup2 [hereinafter referred to as NCCAM, *Complementary medicine*].

43. The citation is to Bonnie O'Connor et al., Defining and describing complementary and alternative medicine, *Alternative Therapies in Health & Medicine, 3,* 2, 49 (1997).

44. Wayne B. Jonas, Policy, the public, and priorities in alternative medicine research, *Annals of the American Academy of Political and Social Sciences, 583,* 29, 33 (2002).

45. Eisenberg et al., Trends, note 2.

46. NCCAM, *Complementary medicine,* note 42.

47. Ralph Snyderman and Andrew Weil, Integrative medicine: Bringing medicine back to its roots, *Archives of Internal Medicine, 162,* 395, 396 (2002).

48. Ibid.

49. Kaptchuk and Eisenberg argue that "[u]ntil recently, the medical community has mainly sought to ignore or suppress unconventional healing," but

now has "begun to seek reconciliation with alternative medicine," and may seek a "peaceful and mutually advantageous reconciliation." Kaptchuk and Eisenberg, Varieties I (2001), at 193. Still, the question remains as to whether the medical profession will "seek to absorb . . . therapies that provide marketing advantages," and whether alternative medicine will "remain a distinct option or become assimilated, 'co-opted,' or truly integrated into a new single 'system.' " Ibid. The authors provocatively ask: "Who gets to decide? . . . Does 'integration' mean elimination of pluralism?" Ibid. Compare with Cohen (2003), *Future medicine*, at 102 (note 33) (defining a regulatory goal of integration as, "the larger aim of a world synthesis of medicine, the potential embrace of accumulated knowledge within all global healing traditions from across time and cultures . . . the process of distilling the collective human wisdom regarding health and healing; it is multidisciplinary and revolutionary; it invokes radical combinations of perspectives on science, human purpose, and ultimate questions such as the meaning of human spiritual evolution"). Stephen Straus, the present director of NCCAM, similarly comments concerning CAM integration: "One model that is espoused, perhaps not surprisingly, by some physicians envisions the incorporation of selected CAM practitioners into the existing conventional medical system. In contrast, CAM practitioners, fearing a loss of identity and purpose, argue that CAM and conventional practitioners should work in parallel." Straus, pers. comm. (2001). He envisions a "merger of valuable CAM and conventional approaches into a practice of 'integrative medicine,' in which multiple health care professions work as an interdisciplinary team." Ibid.

50. Snyderman and Weil, note 47.

51. Cohen, *Future medicine*, at 6 (note 33). "The phrase, 'safe, effective, and appropriate' contains inherent disclaimers that presuppose that clinicians, researchers, and regulators are at the beginning stages of working through the mutually acceptable boundaries of integrative health care. Further, the word 'appropriate' lends a qualitative element to the definition." Ibid.

52. Cohen, *Future medicine*, at 30 (note 33). Jonas, in similar fashion, suggests balancing evaluation strategies "between the criteria of internal validity (focused on identifying causal links) and external validity (focused on clarifying impact and utility)." Callahan (2002), page 174, at 131.

53. See, e.g., Wilk, 895 F.2d at 352 (in which the Seventh Circuit found a nationwide conspiracy by the American Medical Association's Committee on Quackery to "eliminate a licensed profession" of chiropractic).

54. See generally Cohen, *Future medicine*, at 258–276 (note 33) (discussing potential role for spiritual care at end of life and possible legal, ethical, and institutional obstacles).

55. See generally ibid., at 27–80 (framing potential ethical dilemmas); see also Karen E. Adams, Michael H. Cohen, Albert R. Jonsen, and David M. Eisenberg, Ethical considerations of complementary and alternative medical therapies in conventional medical settings, *Annals of Internal Medicine, 137,* 660 (2002).

56. Ibid. The language is taken from our grant.

57. The report is available at http://www.usnews.com/usnews/edu/grad/rankings/med

58. Academic Consortium of Health Centers for Integrative Medicine. Retrieved November 19, 2003, from http://www.pcintegrativemedicine.org/links/acadcon.asp

59. Cohen (1998).

60. Ibid.

61. Ibid. at 15, quoting T. Romeyn Beck, A sketch of the legislative provision of the colony and state of New-York, respecting the practice of physic and surgery, *New York Journal of Medicine, 139* (1822).

62. Ibid. at 26–29 (citing cases). The third element, involving receipt of compensation for the healing service, is not a necessary element in all states.

63. Ibid. at 22 (citing cases).

64. Ibid. at 15.

65. Ibid. at 17, 34–35.

66. Ibid. at 17, quoting Richard H. Shryock, *Medical Licensing in America, 1650–1965.* Baltimore: Johns Hopkins Press, 1967.

67. Ibid. at 34–35 (citing sources). For a seminal critique of licensure, see Walter Gelhorn, The abuse of occupational licensing, *University of Chicago Law Review, 44,* 6 (1976).

68. See Cohen, *Future Medicine,* at 86–87 (note 33).

69. See Cohen (1998), at 35 (citing cases).

70. See, e.g., 2002 Cal. Stat. 820, enacting Cal. Bus. & Prof. Code §§ 2053.5, 2053.6 (also stating the purpose of the legislation).

71. R.I. Gen. Laws § 23-74-1(3). The statute provides that "unlicensed health care practices" do not include

surgery, X-ray radiation, prescribing, administering, or dispensing legend drugs and controlled substances, practices that invade the human body by puncture of the skin, setting fractures, any practice included in the practice of dentistry, the manipulation or adjustment of articulations of joints, or the spine, also known as chiropractic medicine . . . , the healing art of acupuncture . . . , or practices that are permitted under [two other, specific statutes].

72. Ibid. at § 23-74-1(4)(d).

73. Ibid. at § 23-74-1(4).

74. See Cohen, *Future Medicine,* at 29–31 (note 33) (citing cases describing legal action against the nonlicensed CAM provider), and ibid. at 47–55 (citing cases describing legal action against the licensed CAM provider).

75. Cal. Bus. & Prof. Code §2053.5(a) (2002). Retrieved August 4, 2003 from http://www.leginfo.ca.gov/cgi-bin/displaycode?section=bpc&group=02001-03000&file=2050-2079

76. R.I. Gen. Laws § 23-74-4(2). When therapies necessarily involve healing touch, such contact may be more ambiguous than the present statutory language allows. See Cohen (2003), *Future medicine,* at 167–211 (note 33).

77. Ibid. at § 23-74-4(6).

78. Cal. Bus. & Prof. Code §2053.5(a) (2002). Retrieved August 4, 2003 from http://www.leginfo.ca.gov/cgi-bin/displaycode?section=bpc&group=02001-03000&file=2050-2079

79. Cohen (1998), at 39–40.

80. Ibid. at 40–44 (citing statutes).

81. Ibid. at 39.

82. Ibid. at 68–69 (citing cases).

83. Ibid. at 47–49 (citing Matter of Stockwell, 622 P.2d 910 (Wash. App. 1981); Foster v. Georgia Bd. of Chiropractic Examiners, 359 S.E.2d 877 (Ga. 1987)).

84. Ibid.

85. Again, the medical licensing statutes do not seem to make a distinction between the narrower notion of curing, and the broader realm of healing (the latter implying a restored psychosocial and spiritual wholeness).

86. A similar issue arises in trying to conceptualize distinctions between structure–function claims, which are permissible for dietary supplement labels under the Dietary Supplements Health Education Act of 1994, and disease claims, which are impermissible, and bring the supplement in question within the definition of a "drug." See Cohen (1998), at 81 (citing sources). Structure–function claims describe the role of a nutrient or dietary ingredient intended to affect the structure and function in human beings (for example, "saw palmetto maintains prostate health"); whereas disease claims link the dietary supplement to the diagnosis, mitigation, cure, or treatment of a disease (for example, "saw palmetto cures prostate cancer"). Cohen, *Beyond Complementary Medicine*, at 114 (note 32).

87. Cohen (1998), at 109–110.

88. Ibid., at 87 (citing statutes).

89. Alaska Stat. § 08.64.32(a)(8)(A) (2002).

90. Colo. Rev. Stat. § 12-36-117 (2002). Additional statutes are collected at Health Lobby, Health Freedom States. Retrieved August 11, 2003 from http://www.healthlobby.com/statelaw.html

91. See Cohen (1998), at 92–95 (discussing some differences among statutes).

92. Federation of State Medical Boards, Model Guidelines for the Use of Complementary and Alternative Medical Therapies in Medical Practice, Section I. Preamble (April 2002). Retrieved August 11, 2003 from www.fsmb.org

93. United Arab Emirates, Ministerial Resolution No. 600 of 2001 Establishing the Complementary and Alternative Medicine Section.

94. United Arab Emirates, Ministerial Resolution No. 444 of 2006 Regulating the Practice of Complementary (Alternative) Medicine.

95. M. H. Cohen, Medical freedom legislation: Illusory progress? *Alternative and Complementary Therapies*, Vol. 11, 97–101 (2006).

96. 660 N.Y.S.2d 665, 668 (N.Y. Sup. 1997).

97. Ibid. The decision was affirmed, but modified on appeal to vacate the punitive damages award, 673 N.Y.S.2d 685 (App Div. 1998).

98. See Cohen (1998), at 58–59, 62–63 (citing cases, and discussing the potential application of these defenses to use of CAM therapies).

99. Moore v. Baker, 1991 U.S. Dist. LEXIS 14712, at *11 (S.D. Ga., Sept. 5, 1991), aff'd, 989 F.2d 1129 (11th Cir. 1993).

100. 2003 Tenn. App. LEXIS 226.
101. Jones v. Batherson, 2000 Conn. Super. LEXIS 1706.
102. Cohen, Medical freedom legislation, note 95.
103. Credentials Review and Privileging: Questions and Answers for Ambulatory Care, *Comprehensive Accreditation Manual for Hospitals* (JCAHO, 1999).
104. Ibid.
105. Ibid. MS.5.14 (JCAHO).
106. JCAHO (1999), note 103.
107. Eisenberg et al. (2002) page 174. Hospitals can use various national databases to discover whether practitioners have been disciplined. A major database is the National Practitioner Databank (NPDB), a national register of physicians, dentists, and other health care practitioners, established by the federal government. The NPDB "gathers information about practitioners' professional competence and conduct from different regulating organizations for release to eligible entities. NPDB information includes adverse actions against practitioners' clinical privileges, licensure, and professional society memberships. It also gives information about medical malpractice payments." This and related information can be found at www.credentialinfo.com/cred/dbintros/databank/npdb.cfm. The chiropractic profession has its own interjurisdictional chiropractic board action database, called CIN-BAD, which is run by the Federation of Chiropractic Licensing Boards. See www.flcb.org
108. Eisenberg et al. (2002).
109. Ibid.
110. See Cohen (1998), at 36–37 (distinguishing mandatory licensure, title licensure (or "permissive certification"), and registration.
111. See Alan Dumoff, Malpractice liability of alternative/complementary health care providers: A view from the trenches, *Alternative and Complementary Therapies, 1*(4), 248 and *1*(5), 333 (1995).
112. Cf. Bart Nooteboo. *Learning and innovation in organizations and economies*. Oxford: Oxford University Press, 2001.
113. W. Richard Scott, Martin Ruef, Peter J. Mendel, and Carol A. Caronna, *Institutional change and healthcare organizations: From professional dominance to managed care*. Chicago: The University of Chicago Press, 2000.
114. Barbara Wejnert, Integrating models of diffusion of innovations: A conceptual framework, *Annual Review of Sociology, 28*, 297–326 (2002).
115. Harriet Zuckerman, The sociology of science. In Neil K. Smelser (ed.), *Handbook of sociology*, pp. 511–574. Newbury Park, CA, 1988; Steven Shapin, Here and everywhere: Sociology of scientific knowledge, *Annual Review of Sociology, 21*, 289–321 (1995).
116. Karin Knorr Cetina, *The manufacture of knowledge: An essay on the constructivist and contextual nature of science*. Oxford: Pergamon Press, 1981; Karin Knorr Cetina, *Epistemic cultures: How the sciences make knowledge*. Cambridge, MA: Harvard University Press, 1999; Bruno Latour, *Science in action: How to follow scientists and engineers through society*. Cambridge, MA: Harvard University Press, 1987.

117. Donald W. Light, Role protection in an era of accountability: The case of the medical profession. In Judith R. Blau and Norman Goodman (eds.), *Social roles and social institutions: Essays in honor of Rose Laub Coser*, pp. 227–239. Boulder, CO: Westview, 1995.

118. Mark Schlesinger, A loss of faith: The sources of reduced political legitimacy for the American medical profession, *The Milbank Quarterly 80*, 2, 185–235 (2002).

119. Ruggie, Marginal to Mainstream (note 12).

120. The Web site is http://www.imconsortium.org/

121. The Consortium maintains a current list of member schools at http://www .imconsortium.org/cahcim/members/home.html

122. American Hospital Association. *Complementary and Alternative Medicine Survey*, (note 25).

123. Across the IHCs, these three positions—center director, medical director, clinical director—may be occupied by one, two or, theoretically, three persons. Some of the larger centers also have directors for research and education programs, as well as for financial and development functions.

124. Cohen, *Beyond complementary medicine* (note 32); Cohen, *Future medicine* (note 33).

125. W. C. Meeker and S. Haldeman, Chiropractics: A profession at the crossroads of mainstream and alternative medicine, *Annals of Internal Medicine, 136*, 3, 216–227 (2002).

126. J. Jacobs, E. H. Chapman, and D. Crothers, Patient characteristics and practice patterns of physicians using homeopathy, *Archives of Family Medicine, 7* (Nov/Dec 1998).

127. Cohen, *Complementary and alternative medicine*, (note 33).

128. Workshop on Alternative Medicine, *Alternative Medicine: Expanding Medical Horizons. A Report to the National Institute of Health on Alternative Systems and Practices in the United States*. Washington, DC: U.S. Government Printing Office, 1995, xliv–xlv.

129. American Hospital Association. *Complementary and Alternative Medicine Survey*, note 25.

130. White House Commission on Complementary and Alternative Medicine Policy, "Final Report," March 2002, www.whccamp.hbs.gov (February 2004). Insurance companies in the United States presently reimburse only about 10% of the money spent by consumers on CAM; K. R. Pelletier and J. A. Astin, Integration and reimbursement of complementary and alternative medicine by managed care and insurance providers, *Alternative Therapies, 8*, 1, 38–48 (2002); D. Stewart, J. Weeks, and S. Bent, Utilization, patient satisfaction, and cost implications of acupuncture, massage, and naturopathic medicine offered as covered health benefits, *Alternative Therapies, 7*, 4, 66–70 (2001); Landmark Healthcare, Inc., *The Landmark Report II on HMOs and Alternative Care: 1999 Nationwide Study of Alternative Care*. Sacramento, CA: Landmark Healthcare, 1999.

131. Interestingly, one national survey found that half of the HMOs in its sample thought that CAM added to their total health care costs and only about 20% thought it reduced costs. *The Landmark Report II*, note 3.

132. See Joint Commission on Accreditation of Healthcare Organizations. Dictionary of Health Care Terms, Organizations, And Acronyms (1998); Joint Commission on Accreditation of Healthcare Organizations, Credentialing and Privileging (available on-line at www.jacho.org/standard/faq/ltc_credandpriv.html).

133. Barry R. Furrow, Timothy L. Greaney, Sandra H. Johnson, Timothy S. Jost, Robert L. Schwartz, *Health law*, §§ 4-5 to 4-8, at 96–102 (St. Paul, MN: West Publishing Co., 1995). In addition to being required to comply with their own medical staff bylaws, hospitals must meet constitutional due process requirements in credentialing procedures: "The denial, revocation or limitation of staff privileges is ordinarily viewed as deprivation of a property interest." Ibid. at 96–97. Hospitals are also subject to federal and state antidiscrimination statutes, however, which may apply to both employment and staff privileges decisions. Ibid. at 102 (citing sources).

134. Eisenberg et al., *Credentialing* (2002), page 174, at 968. The relative number of states licensing a given provider does not necessarily correlate with the prevalence of such providers nationwide. As of 1999, there were 2,558,874 registered nurses and 684,605 licensed medical doctors in the United States, as compared with 250,000 massage therapists, 185,000 pharmacists, 70,000 chiropractors, and 1,400 naturopathic doctors. Ibid. Interestingly, there were 125 accredited medical schools, 16 accredited chiropractic schools, 4 accredited naturopathy schools, 37 accredited acupuncture schools (and 72 unaccredited). Ibid., at 969. Of the most widely licensed CAM professions—chiropractic, acupuncture, massage therapy, and naturopathy—massage therapy has the greatest proliferation of professional membership and accrediting organizations and has 81 accredited and 990 unaccredited massage therapy schools. Ibid.

135. See generally Cohen (1998), at 39–55 (describing scope of practice variations for chiropractors, naturopathic physicians, acupuncturists, and massage therapists.)

136. Ibid. (citing statutes).

137. Ibid., at 46.

138. Ibid. at 108–109. Scope of practice is controversial even within biomedical care, because the "jurisdictional claims of each profession may overlap." Furrow et al., *Health law*, at 62 (note 133). For example, "the 'practice of medicine' and the 'practice of nursing' can involve the same functions." Ibid. Such "interprofessional 'territorial' disputes' have occurred . . . among other health providers as well: for example, radiologists and chiropractors . . . and nurses and physician assistants." Ibid. at 68 (citing cases). As a result, joint professional or interprofessional boards have been created in some states for some professions. See ibid. at 68–69 (citing sources).

139. 622 P.2d 910 (Wash. Ct. App. 1981).

140. Ibid., at 914.

141. See Cohen (1998), at 46. The reason is that the definitions of "practicing medicine," in most state licensing statutes, are drafted and interpreted sufficiently broadly to capture such situations. See ibid. at 26–33.

142. Once scope of practice boundaries are set, there may be jurisdictional turfs between the integrative care team when practice boundaries overlap. For example, conflicts can arise between massage therapists, physical therapists, and chiropractors over "the exclusivity of hydrotherapy, recommendations for exercise, and certain kinds of tissue manipulation." Eisenberg et al., *Credentialing* (2002), at 969.

143. In other words, the question is whether CAM therapies have been "assimilated, 'co-opted,' or truly integrated into a new single 'system.' " Kaptchuk and Eisenberg, Varieties I (2001), at 193.

144. Interestingly, at this center, the janitorial services were called "integrated services," so the center could not denote its practices as "integrative medicine."

145. Ironically, increasing rigor of quality assurance through tighter credentialing (and risk management) mechanisms can also result in an undesirable increase in bureaucracy and loss of the holistic vision of many CAM therapies. Eisenberg et al., *Credentialing* (2002), at 971.

146. M. H. Cohen, A. Hrbek, R. Davis, S. Schachter, K. J. Kemper, E. W. Boyer, and D. M. Eisenberg, Emerging credentialing practices, malpractice liability policies, and guidelines governing complementary and alternative medical practices and dietary supplements recommendations: A descriptive study of 19 integrative health care centers in the U.S., *Archives of Internal Medicine, 165,* 289–295 (2005).

147. M. H. Cohen, L. Sandler, A. Hrbek, R. B. Davis, and D. M. Eisenberg, Policies pertaining to complementary and alternative medical therapies in a random sample of 39 academic health centers, *Alternative Therapies in Health & Medicine, 11,* 1, 36–40 (2005).

148. Anne Nedrow, Status of credentialing alternative providers within a subset of U.S. academic health centers, *Journal of Alternative and Complementary Medicine, 12,* 3, 329–335 (2006).

149. M. H. Cohen, Harmonizing the cacophony: Commentary on status of credentialing alternative providers within a subset of U.S. academic health centers, *Journal of Alternative and Complementary Medicine, 12,* 3, 337–339 (2006).

150. The grid is adapted from a fuller chart in Michael H. Cohen and David M. Eisenberg, Potential physician malpractice liability associated with complementary/integrative medical therapies, *Annals of Internal Medicine, 136,* 596, 597 (2002). That chart was adapted for patients in a cover story entitled, The Science of Alternative Medicine in *Newsweek* (Dec. 2, 2002).

151. This analysis is presented in greater depth, with clinical examples, in Cohen and Eisenberg, ibid.

152. Ibid., at 597–599.

153. Case examples are included together with the framework, slightly modified, in M. H. Cohen and D. Rosenthal, Legal issues in integrative oncology. In M. P. Mumber (ed.), *Integrative oncology: Principles and practice,* pp. 101–120. Oxford: Taylor and Francis Publishing, 2006.

154. R. Schouten and M. H. Cohen, Legal issues in integration of complementary therapies into cardiology. In W. H. Frishman, M. I. Weintraub, and

M. S. Micozzi (eds.), *Complementary and integrative therapies for cardio-vascular disease*, pp. 20–55. New York and London: Elsevier, 2004.

155. M. H. Cohen and K. J. Kemper, Complementary therapies in pediatrics: A legal perspective. *Pediatrics, 115*, 774–780, 2005; M. H. Cohen, K. J. Kemper, L. Stevens, D. Hashimoto, and J. Gilmour, Pediatric use of complementary therapies: ethical and policy choices. [Electronic pages] *Pediatrics, 116*, e568–e575 (2005).

156. Ibid., at 599–600.

157. This formulation is from Studdert et al., Medical malpractice, at 1614 (note 32).

158. Cohen and Eisenberg (2002), at 601.

159. Cohen (1998), at 68–72 (citing cases).

160. Cohen (1998), at 72.

161. See P. C. Walker, Evolution of a policy disallowing the use of alternative therapies in a health system, *American Journal of Health Policy, 57*, 21, 1984 (2000).

162. See Faass (2001), page 175, 41–114 (discussing practical aspects of strategic planning within the health care institution considering integration of CAM therapies).

163. See, e.g., Dona J. Reese and Mary-Ann Sontag, Successful interprofessional collaboration on the hospice team, *Health & Social Work, 26*, 3, 167 (2001) suggesting that physicians may view the "holistic approach" inherent in hospice philosophy as ancillary to medicine, while social workers may lack training and sensitivity concerning medical expertise and values, and thereby be unable to successfully collaborate "across the cultural boundary that exists between professions." According to the authors, barriers include "lack of knowledge of the expertise of other professions, role blurring, conflicts arising from differences among professions in values and theoretical base, negative team norms, client stereotyping, and administrative issues."

164. One idiosyncratic response was from a center that indicated it had decided to limit hours clinicians can offer services, because of concerns about "potential boundary violations" by clinicians. Another center indicated that, with respect to concern for liability, "nothing jumps out. [We have had] no lawsuits or issues . . . [and] no claims, quality of care issues were raised. The hospital had no particular concerns."

165. The medical director explained that once he designed credentialing guidelines for CAM providers

Legal counsel . . . came up with questions regarding contraindications, record-keeping requirements, when are these "patients" or not. We came up with this as a solution: the person is a "patient" if you treat them for a medical condition (like yoga for back pain; cancer; or heart disease). If they're a patient, we have them physician-referred so MDs can screen for contraindications. Their physician must approve it and then refer them to us for that provider. Legal counsel dealt with liability issues this way: They have the MD refer the patient to our CAM provider, and that puts the burden on the MD to screen for contraindications and for other possible underlying medical conditions.

166. The head of risk management for the center, a lawyer, commented:

Hospital counsel was involved in the early stages, but ultimately the details of the protocols she delegated to our ad hoc committee. We have a lawyer on our credentials committee; but lawyers only get involved if there's a question of taking disciplinary action and how do we keep inside the rules, bylaws. I oversee the third-party claims administrators, who run our claims, and our defense counsel.

167. This strategy is arguably the most critical. See Cohen and Eisenberg, Potential physician malpractice, at 601 (note 150).

168. As of 2001, only 12 states of those that licensed non-MD acupuncturists had some statutory requirement of prior written authorization, referral, or supervision. Barbara B. Mitchell, *Acupuncture and oriental medicine laws*, 152–157 and Table 7 (Washington, DC: National Acupuncture Foundation, 2002).

169. Another center reported on energy healing practices as follows:

Almost everybody who practiced in the clinic did energy healing: for example, the acupuncturist did Mari-El and Reiki and Qi Gong; nurses did healing touch. We didn't credential for it. We just looked broadly at how we interpreted the scope of practice. We have a transplant pulmonologist who has let energy healers come in during procedures to remove the spirit of the old lung that is being transplanted. [We are] open to shamanistic practices.

The director clarified that many patients "are requesting energy work pre-operatively as well as intra-operatively," but that offering this was limited by a decision made by the anesthesia department that only employees of the institution could be in the operating room.

170. Wendy A. Weiger, Michael Smith, Heather Boon, Mary Ann Richardson, Ted J. Kaptchuk, and David M. Eisenberg, Advising patients who seek complementary and alternative medical therapies for cancer, *Annals of Internal Medicine, 137,* 889 (2002). The grid is adapted from Cohen and Eisenberg (2002), and adds to that framework suggestions for what kind and level of evidence (e.g., number of randomized controlled trials or other evidence) would be necessary for a given therapy to fit within a given region of the framework.

171. See Barbara B. Mitchell, *Acupuncture and oriental medicine laws* (Washington, DC: National Acupuncture Foundation, 2002).

172. Cohen et al., Emerging credentialing practices (note 146); Cohen et al., Policies (note 147).

173. See Eisenberg, Advising (note 38).

174. David M. Eisenberg, Ronald C. Kessler, Maria I. Van Rompay, Ted Kaptchuk, S. A. Wilkey, S. Appel et al., Perceptions about use and non-disclosure

of complementary and alternative therapies: Results from a national survey, *Annals of Internal Medicine, 135*, 344 (2001).

175. Ibid.
176. See generally The President's Commission for the Study of Ethical Problems in Medicine and Biomedical Research, *Making health care decisions: The social and ethical issues of informed consent in the patient–practitioner relationship* (Washington, DC: U.S. Government Printing Office, 1982).
177. Schloendorff v. Society of New York Hospital, 105 N.E.2d 92, 93 (1914).
178. See Edzard E. Ernst and Michael H. Cohen, Informed Consent in Complementary and Alternative Medicine, *Archives of Internal Medicine, 161*, 19, 2288 (2001).
179. Ibid. (citing sources).
180. Ibid.
181. Moore v. Baker, 1991 U.S. Dist. LEXIS 14712, at *11 (S.D. Ga., Sept. 5, 1991), *aff'd*, 989 F.2d 1129 (11th Cir. 1993).
182. National Institutes of Health, NIH Consensus Conference: Acupuncture, *Journal of the American Medical Association, 280*, 17, 1518 (1998); S. J. Bigos, O. R. Bowyer, R. G. Braen, K. Brown, R. Deyo, and Scott Haldeman, *Acute low back problems in adults: Clinical practice guideline* (Number 14). Agency for Health Care Policy and Research, Rockville, MD: U.S. Dept. Health and Human Services, 1994; NIH Technology Assessment Statement, *Integration of behavioral and relaxation approaches into the treatment of chronic pain and insomnia*. Bethesda, MD: National Institutes of Health, 1995.
183. S. C. Piscitelli, A. H. Surstein, D. Chaitt, R. M. Alfaro, and J. Falloon, Indinavir concentrations and St. John's wort, *Lancet, 355*, 547 (2000).
184. M. H. Cohen, Negotiating integrative medicine: a framework for provider–patient conversations. *Negotiation Journal, 30*, 3, 409–433 (2004).
185. Adams et al., Ethical considerations (note 55).
186. Ibid.
187. Ibid.
188. *Complementary and alternative medicine in the United States* (Institute of Medicine of the National Academies) National Academies Press: Washington, DC, 2005.
189. Ibid., p. 172.
190. Ibid., p. 8.
191. Cohen, Harmonizing (note 149), quoting M. H. Cohen, *Legal issues in integrative medicine*. Washington, DC: NAF Publications, 2005.
192. E. E. Ernst, M. H. Cohen, and J. Stone, Ethical problems arising in evidence-based complementary and alternative medicine, *Journal of Medical Ethics, 30*, 156–159 (2004); K. Kemper and M. H. Cohen, Ethics in complementary medicine: New light on old principles, *Contemporary Pediatrics, 21*, 3, 61–72 (2004).
193. Dietary Supplements Health Education Act, 103 P.L. 417; 108 Stat. 4325; 1994.
194. Pub. L. No. 103-417, 108 Stat. 4325, 21 U.S.C. § § 301 et seq. (1994).
195. U. S. Food and Drug Administration, Center for Food Safety and Applied

Nutrition, Overview of Dietary Supplements. (Retrieved from vm.cfsan
.fda.gov/~dms/ds-oview.html). The FDA's recent proposed rule regarding
good manufacturing practices for dietary supplements is found on its Web
site at www.fda.gov/bbs/topics/NEWS/dietarysupp

196. Alan Dumoff has written a number of helpful articles in this arena. See
Alan Dumoff, State medical board prohibitions on physician sale of supplements: A looming issue, *Physician Consult* (Aug. 2000); Alan Dumoff,
Medical board prohibitions against physician supplements sales, *Alternative and Complementary Therapies, 6*, 4, 226 (2000). As suggested, other
rules, such as those prohibiting so-called kickbacks and self-referrals, also
may apply. See generally Alan Dumoff, Regulating professional relationships: Kickback and self-referral restrictions on collaborative practice, *Alternative and Complementary Therapies, 6*, 1, 41 (2000); see also Alan
Dumoff, Understanding the Kassenbaum-Kennedy Health Care Act:
Addressing legitimate concerns and irrational fears, *Alternative and Complementary Therapies, 3*, 4, 309; Alan C. Dumoff, Legislation versus self-
regulation in the somatic practices field: Comments from the editor,
Alternative and Complementary Therapies, 3, 3, 220 (1997). See also L. K.
Campbell, C. J. Ladenheim, R. P. Sherman, and L. Sportelli, *Professional
Chiropractic Practice: Ethics, Business, Jurisprudence and Risk Management*, pp. 53–90, 157–213. Fincastle, VA: Health Services Publication,
2001 (discussing broader legal concerns applicable to CAM providers such
as chiropractors).

197. Some of the suggestions and material in this chapter were given as part
of a talk by Michael H. Cohen, entitled "Regulatory and Legal Issues Concerning Herbal Therapies and Dietary Supplements," at a conference entitled, "Herbal Therapies and Other Dietary Supplements: What the
Practicing Physician, Pharmacist or Nurse Needs to Know" (sponsored by
Harvard Medical School and the University of California, San Francisco),
2004.

198. N.J. Bd. Of Med. Examiners, Regulation 45.9-22.11.

199. See, e.g., Charell, 660 N.Y.S. 2d at 668.

200. See, e.g., Adrian Fugh-Berman, Herb–Drug Interactions, *Lancet, 355*, 134
(2000); Edzard E. Ernst, Second Thoughts About Safety of St. John's Wort,
Lancet, 354, 2014 (1999).

201. See Council on Ethical and Judicial Affairs AMA, American Medical Association, Sale of non-health-related goods from physicians' offices, *Journal of the American Medical Association, 280*, 563 (1998).

202. The interviewee reported having had some satisfaction regarding quality
assurance with a specific manufacturer of Chinese herbs from Taiwan, noting: "the . . . tests they perform show a low level of adulterants and con-
tamination in their products."

203. Such disclosure arguably respects the patient's autonomy interest and is
ethically supportable. See generally Karen E. Adams, Michael H. Cohen,
Albert R. Jonsen, David M. Eisenberg, Ethical considerations of complementary and alternative medical therapies in conventional medical settings,
Annals of Internal Medicine, 137, 660 (2002) (framing ethical perspectives).

204. This liability management approach is recommended in Cohen and Eisenberg (2002).

205. This is similar to the notion of manufacturers being allowed, under the DSHEA, to make structure-function but not disease claims. See ibid.

206. O. Hatch, *Square peg: Confessions of a citizen senator*, pp. 81–95. New York: Basic Books, 2002.

207. L. Bjerkenstedt et al., Hypericum extract and fluoxetine in mild to moderate depression: a randomized, placebo-controlled multi-center study in outpatients, *European Archives of Psychiatry and Clinical Neuroscience, 255*, 40–47 (2005).

208. J. P. Kelly et al., Recent trends in use of herbal and other natural products, *Archives of Internal Medicine, 165*, 281–286 (2005).

209. M. Hardy, Review of recent clinical trials involving herbal supplements. In *Natural supplements: An evidence-based update*, pp. 429–441. San Diego: University of California, 2006.

210. Hypericum Depression Trial Study Group, Effect of *Hypericum perforatum* (St John's wort) in major depressive disorder: A randomized controlled trial, *Journal of the American Medical Association, 287*, 14, 1807–1814 (2002).

211. B. Vitiello et al., Hyperforin plasma level as a marker of treatment adherence in the NIH Hypericum Depression Trial, *Journal of Clinical Psychopharmacology, 25*, 243–249 (2005).

212. M. Fava et al., A double-blind, randomized trial of St John's wort, fluoxetine and placebo in major depressive disorder, *Journal of Clinical Psychopharmacology, 25*, 441–447 (2005).

213. M. Gastpar et al., Efficacy and tolerability of hypericum extract in long-term treatment with a once-daily dosage in comparison with sertraline, *Pharmacopsychiatry, 38*, 78–86 (2005).

214. A. Szegedi et al., Acture treatment of moderate to severe depression with hypericum extract (SJW): Randomized controlled double-blind non inferiority trial versus paroxetine, *British Medical Journal, 330*, 503 (2005); Erratum in *British Medical Journal, 330*, 759 (2005).

215. K. Linde and M. Berner, St John's wort comparison studies and meta-analysis, *British Journal of Psychiatry, 186*, 99–107 (2005).

216. P. R. Solomon, F. Adams, A. Silver, J. Zimmer, and R. DeVeaux, Gingko for memory enhancement: A randomized controlled trial. *Journal of the American Medical Association, 288*, 7, 835–840 (2002).

217. P. A. De Smet, Herbal remedies, *New England Journal of Medicine, 347*, 2046–2056 (2002).

218. Jiang et al., Effect of gingko and ginger on the pharmacokinetics and pharmacodynamics of warfarin in healthy subjects, *British Journal of Clinical Pharmacology, 50*, 425–432 (2005).

219. D. Loew and W. Gaus, Kava-Kava. Tragödie einer Fehlbeurteilung. *Zeitschriff Phytotherapie, 23*, 267–281 (2002).

220. W. M. Lee, Acetaminophen and the US Acute Liver Failure Study Group: Lowering the risks of hepatic failure, *Hepatology, 40*, 1, 6–9 (2004).

221. J. Gruenwald, C. Mueller, and J. Skrabal, Kava ban highly questionable: A brief summary of the main scientific findings presented in the "In Depth Investigation on EU Member States Market Restrictions on Kava Products," *Seminars in Integrative Medicine, 1*, 4, 199–210 (2003).

222. *Nutrition Business Journal*, February 2002.

223. M. Sovak, A. L. Seligson, M. Konas, M. Hajduch, M. Dolezal, M. Machala, et al., Herbal composition PC-SPES for management of prostate cancer: Identification of active principles, *JNCI: Journal of the National Cancer Institute, 94*, 1275–1281 (2002).

224. U.S. Customs Service and Food and Drug Administration. *U.S. Customs Service and Food and Drug Administration Uncover Dumping Scheme Involving Contaminated Honey Imports from China.* Food and Drug Administration Office of Public Affairs; August 28, 2002. Retrieved February 2006 from http://www.fda.gov/bbs/topics/NEWS/2002/NEW00831.html

225. K. M. Fairfield and R. H. Fletcher, Vitamins for chronic disease prevention in adults: Scientific evidence, *Journal of the American Medical Association, 287*, 3116–3126 (2002).

226. R. H. Fletcher and K. M. Fairfield, Vitamins for chronic disease prevention in adults: Clinical applications, *Journal of the American Medical Association, 287*, 3127–3129 (2002).

227. Eisenberg et al., Trends, note 2.

228. M. H. Cohen and D. M. Eisenberg, Potential physician malpractice liability associated with complementary and integrative medical therapies, *Annals of Internal Medicine, 136*, 596–603 (2002).

229. Cohen (2003), *Future Medicine*, pp. 93–99 (note 33), citing Abraham Maslow, *Toward a psychology of being*, 2nd ed., p. 114. New York: Van Nostrand, 1968.

230. Testimony of Donald Novey, MD before the Institute of Medicine Committee on Use of Complementary and Alternative Therapies by the American Public, September 2003. Available at www.iom.edu\cam

Index